Making Life More Liv...

Simple adaptations for living at home after vision loss

Revised by Maureen A. Duffy

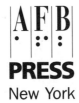

PRESS
New York

9\02

First edition © 1983
Revised edition © 2002

Library of Congress Cataloging-in-Publication Data
Duffy, Maureen A.
  Making life more livable : simple adaptations for living at home after vision loss / revised by Maureen A. Duffy.– Rev. ed.
      p. cm.
Rev. ed. of: Making life more livable / by Irving R. Dickman. c1983.
Includes bibliographical references and index.
    ISBN 0-89128-387-0 (alk. paper)
  1. Aged people with visual disabilities–Rehabilitation. 2. Self-help devices for people with disabilities. I. Dickman, Irving R. Making life more livable. II. Title.
    HV1597.5 .D83 2002
    649.8–dc21

                                                        2002018252

The American Foundation for the Blind—the organization to which Helen Keller devoted more than 40 years of her life—is a national nonprofit whose mission is to eliminate the inequities faced by the 10 million Americans who are blind or visually impaired.

It is the policy of the American Foundation for the Blind to use in the first printing of its books acid-free paper that meets the ANSIZ39.48 Standard. The infinity symbol that appears above indicates that the paper in this printing meets that standard.

Contents

1

Living Independently with Vision Loss

Older People: Myths and Reality

Like everyone else, people in the later years of life are very much distinct individuals. We all have different life histories, personal characteristics, occupations, activities, and preferences, no matter what our age. Contrary to the outdated stereotype of frailty and illness in old age, most older men and women continue to be vibrant, productive, involved members of their families and communities. They continue to pursue their interests and activities and discover new ones; enjoy increased leisure time; and continue to live independent, dynamic lives. As psychologist G. Stanley Hall wrote at age 78, old age can be seen "not as a period of decline and decay," but rather "as a stage of development in which the passions of youth and the efforts of a life career had reached fruition and consolidation."

In fact, given the reality that people today tend to remain vigorous and active far longer than ever before, it is increasingly difficult to determine when "old age" actually begins. Many older people continue to work well into their 80s and beyond, while others may opt for early retirement to pursue a range of educational or leisure interests. Many men and women in their 70s, 80s, and even 90s have no special physical limitations on their daily activities. In other words, it is no longer clear where to place the punctuation mark that signifies the onset of old age.

Older men and women are a dynamic presence in today's society, exerting considerable social, political, and economic influence. The International Center on Longevity, a nonprofit institute that studies aging, located in New York City, projects that within 25 years, in nearly every country in the Northern Hemisphere, one in five persons will be aged 60 or older. The U.S. Bureau of the Census reports that the number of persons aged 65 or older has increased from 25 million in 1980 to 35 million at present and is expected to reach 70 million by 2030. The fastest-growing segment of this population is the 85-and-older age group, whose numbers are expected to nearly double from 4.5 million at present to 8.5 million in 2030. Within this growing population of older adults, most live independently or within family settings in the community. Only 5 percent reside in institutions, such as nursing homes or other long-term-care settings.

One unforeseen by-product of this increased life expectancy, however, is the growing incidence of visual impairments among older persons:

- 70–75 percent of all new cases of visual impairment occur in the 65+ age group.

- Approximately 70 percent of individuals with severe visual impairments are 65 and older.

- The American Foundation for the Blind estimates that 3 million to 3.5 million Americans aged 65+ are severely visually impaired at present, and that this figure will increase to 7.0 million by 2030.

Living Independently with Vision Loss

If you are reading this book, chances are that you have a vision problem—or know someone who does. You may also feel overwhelmed as you deal with vision loss in addition to other changes associated with growing older. However, losing vision does not mean giving up your independence or the activities you enjoy. With a bit of thought and common sense, you can adjust your environment and everyday tasks to make life safer, easier, more enjoyable, and more livable.

Making your home (and your life) more livable doesn't have to be complicated and costly. Many useful adaptations are as simple as installing a brighter lightbulb, opening the curtains to let in more light for reading, or placing a dark sheet of plastic on the kitchen counter to contrast with light-colored foods or dishes. This book focuses on simple, practical, and inexpensive solutions that you can put in place yourself.

When coming to terms with vision loss, it is important to realize that there are no "rules" that fit everyone. Just as every individual is different, no two people have the same type and degree of vision loss; the same lifestyle; the same kind of home; or the same needs, wants, and preferences. Moreover, there are usually several ways to deal with a given situation or problem, and solutions should be tailored to each individual. This book surveys the most common needs of visually impaired older people and offers suggestions that you can put into practice on your own. Specifically, it provides you with information that will help you to

■ learn about normal age-related vision changes and common eye disorders;

■ understand how these vision changes and eye disorders affect everyday activities;

■ evaluate your home for its safety and accessibility;

■ make simple, low-cost, appropriate changes in your environment;

■ find resources for further information and assistance.

You will find the suggestions in this book helpful even if you have only minor vision problems. If you or someone you know has experienced significant vision loss, this book has vital information for you.

Vision and Aging

Any type of change in the way you see can significantly affect your ability to get around safely and independently. By far the major portion of information we receive about the environment is processed through the visual sense; thus, changes in vision can have a substantial impact on our ability not only to receive information but also to analyze it and correctly interpret our surroundings.

To gain a better understanding of vision, it is helpful to think of it as consisting of two distinct components or "systems." The "where" system uses *peripheral vision* to locate objects and avoid obstacles. The "what" system uses *central vision* to recognize and identify objects. Usually, these two systems work together to help you analyze and make sense of the environment: The "where" system detects an object, and the "what" system identifies it.* However, when vision changes affect one or both of these systems, you need to learn to compensate by changing or modifying elements in the environment. It is also important to differentiate between *normal* vision changes that occur in the

---

* These terms were coined by R. McGillivray, in *Aids and Appliances Review: Aids for Elderly Persons with Impaired Vision* (Boston: Carroll Center for the Blind, 1984).

course of aging and severe *eye disorders* that require medical treatment and intervention.

Normal Age-Related Changes in Vision

As people get older, they experience gradual changes in the way they see, as a result of the normal aging process. You are probably familiar with the increased difficulty in reading and seeing things up close that most people begin to experience at about age 40. Other common changes may be less obvious. The following are some significant age-related vision changes:

■ *Decreased color perception.* Distinguishing certain colors becomes more difficult as people get older, which may make it difficult to match outfits, pair socks, sew, play card games, or work on a computer. In particular, it is often hard to distinguish navy blue from brown or black, blue from green or purple; and pink from yellow or pale green.

■ *Reduced contrast sensitivity.* Seeing an object clearly against a background of the same color becomes more difficult. For example, a white plate or coffee mug on a light tablecloth, a brown coffee table against a dark carpet, or a white toothbrush against a white bathroom sink may seem to merge into the background. Greater contrast between the object and the background is necessary for the object to "stand out."

■ *Decreased depth perception.* Judging distances accurately—the height of a step or curb, or the

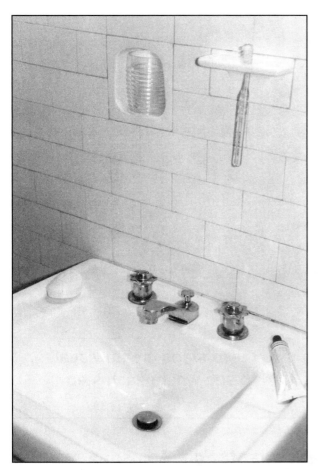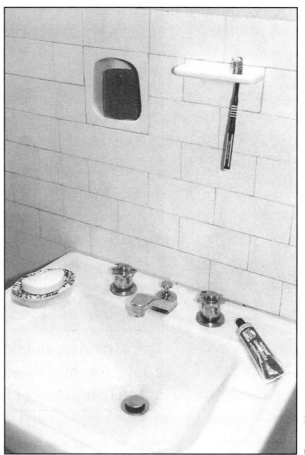

Dave Newman

The white toothbrush and cup *(left)* seem to disappear when placed against the white sink and tiles. It is much easier to see the items when a dark blue cup and toothbrush are used to increase their contrast with the background *(right)*.

depth of a bathtub—requires close attention to safety cues such as color, contrast, and lighting. Shadows and shadow patterns may be incorrectly interpreted as drop–offs or obstacles.

● ***Increased sensitivity to glare.*** Reflected light or bright sunlight outdoors on a sunny day or, for example, in a hallway with highly polished floors may make it increasingly difficult to see the environment clearly.

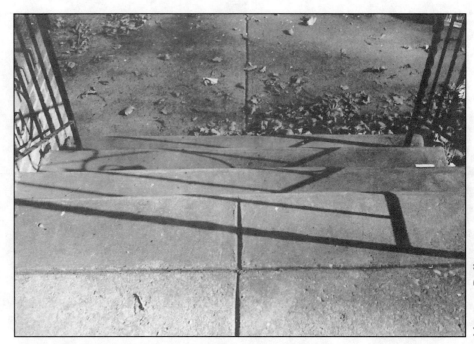

Maureen Duffy

The shadows falling across these steps create visual confusion and make it hard to see where each step actually ends.

- ● *Decreased light-dark adaptation.* Adjusting to changes in lighting levels between bright and dark areas can take significantly longer as one becomes older. Abrupt transitions, such as leaving a dim building lobby and walking outdoors into bright sunlight or entering a darkened movie theater from a brightly lighted concession area, may become more difficult.

- ● *Decreased ability to focus close up.* As the eye muscles that control the switching of focus from far to near begin to lose flexibility, it becomes more difficult to focus on things close up. Performing such everyday activities as reading a newspaper, writing, or sewing usually requires reading glasses to accommodate this change in focus.

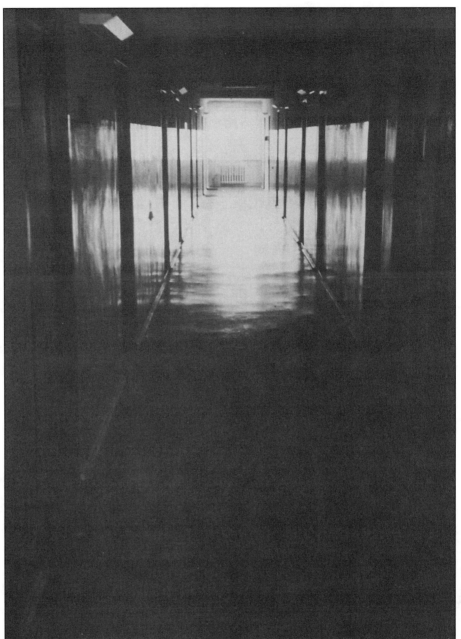

Maureen Duffy

The light from the window reflecting off the shiny floor in this hallway creates glare, which makes it difficult to see details in the environment, including edges between the floor and the walls and any potential safety hazards.

■ ***Increased lighting requirements.*** Most older people need three to four times more light than they did previously to perform certain types of everyday activities. Seeing clearly enough to read,

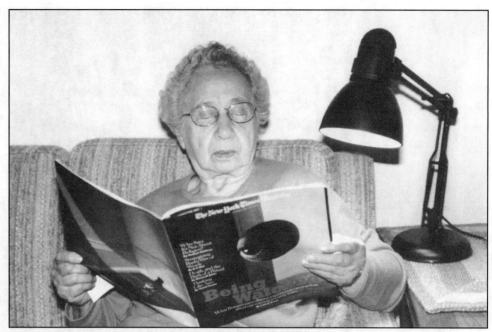

Dave Newman

Bright, high-intensity, or halogen light focused directly on the task makes it easier to see close-up activities such as reading or sewing.

write, sew, knit, or perform home repairs usually requires a brighter, more focused light in addition to reading glasses or bifocals.

Age-Related Eye Disorders

Unlike normal age-related changes in vision, severe *eye disorders* require ongoing treatment from an ophthalmologist, optometrist, or physician. Most of these disorders cause permanent vision loss that cannot be corrected with regular eyeglasses or contact lenses. However, 85 percent to 90 percent of older persons with these age-related eye disorders have some remaining sight—also known as "low vision."

The following are eye disorders that occur most commonly in older people (although children and young adults can experience them as well), along with the types of vision loss they cause and their effect on everyday activities. It is also possible to experience several eye disorders at the same time.

● *Cataracts.* Cataracts are cloudy areas in the lens of the eye. They cause an all-over blurring of both central and peripheral vision, making people, objects, and colors appear hazy and "washed out." This lack of detail makes it difficult to read, tell time, watch television, and walk safely, since depth perception may also be affected. Fortunately, surgery is usually effective in removing cataracts.

● *Diabetic retinopathy.* People with diabetes may develop a condition called diabetic retinopathy, in which the blood vessels of the eye leak or grow abnormally, causing scattered "blind spots." Vision can vary unpredictably from one day to the next, accompanied by both blurring and loss of peripheral vision. This fluctuating vision may interfere with a wide range of everyday activities, including reading, writing, telling time, administering insulin or other medications, and moving about safely indoors and outdoors.

● *Glaucoma.* Glaucoma is characterized by a buildup of fluid in the eye that creates increased pressure. It affects side (or peripheral) vision, creating a "tunnel vision" effect, similar to looking into a tube or narrow tunnel. This loss of side vision makes it difficult to see and avoid objects that are off to the side, near the head, or by the feet.

● ***Macular degeneration.*** Macular degeneration, the most common eye condition among older people, weakens the central portion of the retina (the *macula*), the part of the eye that is responsible for central and color vision. It causes a gray or blank spot directly in the center of the visual field, making it difficult to perform such tasks as reading a book, dialing a telephone, threading a needle, hammering a nail, and seeing faces clearly.

● ***Vision loss resulting from stroke, retinal detachment, brain damage, or trauma.*** Vision loss can also result from a stroke or other event (although these are not, strictly speaking, eye

Most people who have a visual impairment because of an age-related eye disorder still have some vision. These views of the same living room suggest how a person with normal functional vision (**1**) might see a scene and how it might be experienced by individuals with different eye conditions. (**2**) *Cataracts* cause an overall blurring and haziness of vision. (**3**) People with *diabetic retinopathy* can have scattered blind spots, blurring, or loss of side vision that can vary from day to day. (**4**) *Glaucoma* affects side vision, causing a tunnel vision effect. (**5**) *Macular degeneration* leaves a blind spot in the middle of the visual field. (**6**) Some people who have had a *stroke* or severe trauma that affects their vision have distorted vision or lose sight in half the visual field.

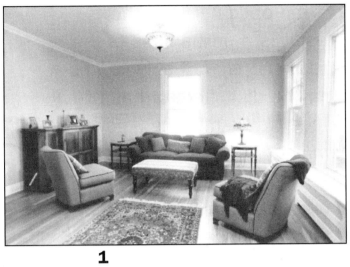

1

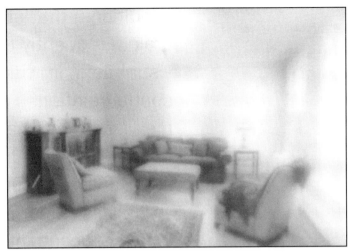

2

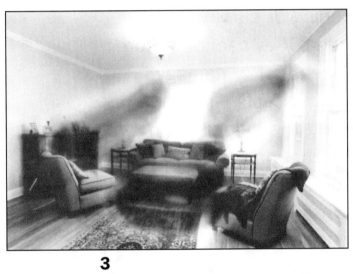

3

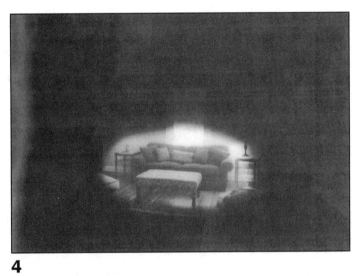

4

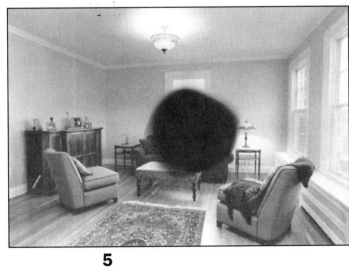

5

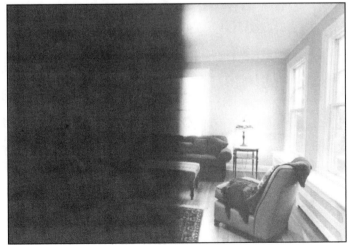

6

conditions) that affects the optic nerve or the brain. Frequently the result is a partial loss of the visual field, in which the perception of objects and spatial relationships may be distorted, or half of the visual field may appear to be missing (known as *hemianopsia* or *hemianopia*). This perceptual distortion can affect reading, writing, dressing, grooming, indoor and outdoor mobility, and most other independent everyday activities.

Most of the time, medical or surgical treatments are effective only in stopping or slowing the progression of the disorder. They cannot restore vision that has already been lost or damaged (although surgery is usually effective in removing cataracts). For this reason, it is helpful to know about special eye care services that help people with low vision, as well as ways of continuing one's daily life and activities with reduced vision.

Maintaining Your Independence after Vision Loss

Low Vision Services

If you have experienced any loss of vision, there are many services and devices that can help you continue to live independently in your own home and community. The place to start is with your eye care professional:

■ An *ophthalmologist* diagnoses and treats eye diseases, in some cases prescribing medications or surgery to improve or prevent the worsening of vision-related conditions.

● An *optometrist* diagnoses eye disorders and prescribes eyeglasses and contact lenses, low vision devices, vision therapy, and medications to treat eye diseases.

If the vision loss cannot be completely corrected and interferes with your everyday living, it is important to schedule a visit with a low vision specialist.

● A *low vision specialist* is either an ophthalmologist or an optometrist who is trained to conduct a special low vision eye examination.

The low vision examination includes a *functional vision assessment* to determine how your specific visual impairment affects your ability to perform everyday activities. The low vision specialist can also determine whether special devices, improved lighting, or other types of vision-related rehabilitation services can help you use your vision more efficiently and effectively. A low vision specialist can recommend and prescribe the following devices and provide information on helpful services:

● *Special optical devices* use lenses to magnify images so that objects or print appear larger to the eye. Examples include magnifiers, pocket-sized telescopes, or closed-circuit televisions.

● *Nonoptical devices and modifications* make changes in the environment or alter objects to make them more easily visible. Improved lighting,

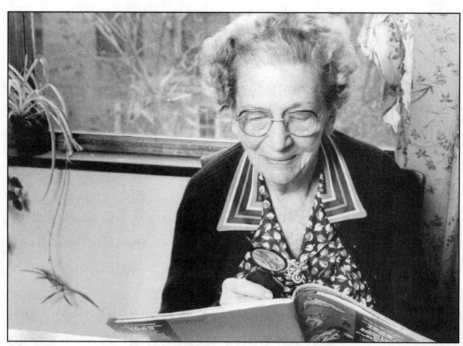

1

Janet Charles

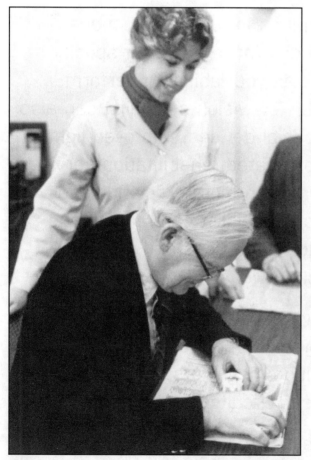

2

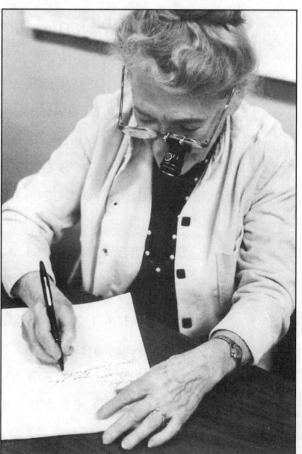

3

Susan Islam

special high-intensity table or floor lamps, large-print reading materials, and greater contrast between objects and the background are examples of nonoptical modifications and devices.

● *Adaptive daily living equipment* includes devices that are designed to make everyday tasks easier to do with little or no vision. Clocks and timers with large numerals, writing guides, needle threaders, large-print or talking watches, and large-print and tactile labels are examples of such equipment.

During the low vision examination, it is important to ask the following questions:

● What is the cause of my vision loss?

● What is my visual acuity (measured eyesight)?

Optical low vision devices use lenses to enlarge the image that reaches the eye. **(1) Handheld magnifiers** work well for a variety of close tasks, such as reading. They are also lightweight and portable. **(2)** Because **stand magnifiers** sit on the page, they hold the lens steady at a fixed distance. Some come with built-in lighting. **(3) Telemicroscopes** allow a person to perform tasks at a more normal distance than do strong reading eyeglasses or magnifiers. This ability can be important when performing tasks that are uncomfortable when done close up, such as viewing a computer screen, knitting, or playing music. Telemicroscopes are mounted on eyeglass frames to leave hands free to engage in various tasks.

Where to Find Help

The simplest way to begin looking for help is to ask your eye care professional for a referral to a low vision specialist and/or an agency that provides vision rehabilitation services. In addition to state agencies, many communities have private agencies that serve people who have experienced vision loss. These agencies provide low vision and independent living or rehabilitation services. Many such organizations may have the word "blind" in their name, but most agencies assist people with varying degrees of vision loss, not just those without any sight. Some agencies have fees for services; others do not.

To find a source of assistance, check your local telephone directory, telephone the American Foundation for the Blind (AFB) at 1-800-232-5463, or write to afbinfo@afb.net. AFB's web site, www.afb.org, contains a complete on-line directory of services. The Resource Guide at the back of this book lists other national organizations that can be contacted for information.

Many adaptive living products that are specially designed to help people with visual impairments carry out their everyday tasks independently are sold through catalogs. The Resource Guide in this book lists some of the most comprehensive catalogs, along with some that specialize in particular types of products.

■ Do I have a loss of peripheral (side) vision?

■ What is the prognosis for my eye condition?

■ Will my condition remain stable, or will I lose more sight?

■ Can I benefit from vision-related rehabilitation training?

■ Am I entitled to special services or benefits?

■ What other resources are available to help me?

Other Vision-Related Rehabilitation Services

Rehabilitation can help people regain self-sufficiency and improve the quality of their lives. *Vision-related rehabilitation services* can help you regain the ability to function independently after vision loss, just as physical therapy can help an individual regain the ability to function after losing the use of a limb. Besides the low vision examination and prescription of devices and modifications, vision-related rehabilitation services include the following:

1. Training in adaptive techniques to restore the ability to function in the following areas:

   ■ Home and personal management skills (such as preparing meals, performing personal care activities such as bathing and grooming, managing money, and labeling medications);

- Communication skills (including the use of readers, tape recorders, braille, large print, computers with screen magnification, writing guides, telephones, and timepieces);

- Independent movement and travel skills (learning to orient yourself in familiar and unfamiliar environments, to ask for assistance from others when appropriate, and to move about using a long white cane or other devices).

2. Individual counseling to help you adjust to vision loss.

3. Support groups that give you the opportunity to talk with others about similar problems and ways to cope.

The types of vision changes described in this chapter can affect how you get around and how you go about your everyday activities. Although a change in vision can involve difficult emotional reactions and adjustments, people who have experienced a loss of vision can continue to go about their lives and activities and remain independent in their own homes. The rest of this book contains information about simple ways to make life in your own home easier and safer. The next chapter discusses how to look at your everyday surroundings to discover where you need to make changes. It also presents some basic principles that will help you make your home safer, better organized, and more livable.

Making Your Environment More Livable: General Principles

Most people have a strong desire to live independently and, even if they have experienced vision loss, to continue living in their own homes. But spouses, family members, and friends are often concerned about a person's ability to live alone when he or she has lost some vision, particularly if the person is elderly. Although some individuals with vision loss may choose relocation or alternative living arrangements in response to concerns about safety and quality of life, it is not the appropriate solution for everyone.

One way to address this situation is to examine your everyday environment carefully and make changes in your surroundings and activities that will help you feel safer, more comfortable, more organized, and more in control of your daily life, despite your vision loss. The first step is to walk through your home and conduct an actual survey of your surroundings (this is sometimes called an *environmental assessment*).

As you review your situation, you might find it helpful to use a checklist like the one at the end of this chapter to make notes about your home. An organized list can help you pay closer attention to your surroundings, including potential problem areas that you might overlook because you've become accustomed to living, working, and moving about in your familiar environment. For example, you might be "making do" with a small table lamp that you have owned for many years, even though your lighting requirements have changed over time; or you may not be aware that the morning sun shining through your uncovered kitchen window is creating distracting glare spots on the floor.

To make this survey as practical as possible, try to think about two general aspects of your home life:

● Your home and immediate surroundings

● Specific everyday activities that you need to do within your home

Remember that examining and changing your home environment and everyday activities are highly individual procedures—there is never only one correct answer or one correct solution. To make *your* home more livable, it is helpful to ask the following questions that are specific to your own daily life and routine:

● How does my vision loss affect my everyday activities?

● What are the basic principles I should consider when assessing my environment at home?

● What safety issues should I consider?

● What types of everyday activities do I need to perform?

● What kinds of simple solutions can I put into place on my own?

● What adaptations should I consider if I have another disability in addition to my vision loss?

These questions are considered throughout the rest of this and the following chapters.

Assessing the Environment: Basic Principles

When you examine your home to see where changes would be helpful, there are several basic elements to consider:

● lighting

● color and contrast

● organization

● texture and touch

● sound

● labels, lettering, and marking

● safety

This chapter explains each of these basic environmental elements and presents general guidelines for making the best use of these elements and examples

(Text continues on page 26)

Basic Principles for Making a Home More Livable for Someone with Vision Loss

Improve Visibility

☑ Provide adequate lighting for the task at hand.

☑ Reduce glare—reflected light from shiny surfaces—that interferes with seeing.

☑ Maximize contrast between objects and their background.

☑ Use bright colors to make objects and edges—such as door frames or moldings along walls—stand out.

☑ Use large- and bold-print reading matter and devices to make maximum use of low vision.

Get Organized!

☑ Organize your belongings into predictable groupings.

☑ Store equipment and supplies near the activity for which they are used.

☑ Always return things to the same place.

☑ Eliminate clutter wherever possible by disposing of unnecessary items and finding places for everything else.

Use Other Senses

☑ Learn to identify places and objects by their feel or sound.

☑ Use adaptive devices that rely on touch or sound, such as a ruler with raised markings or a talking clock.

☑ Minimize background noises to make optimal use of your hearing.

Use Labels

☑ Use appropriate labels to identify items that are hard to distinguish.

☑ Use wide, thick markers to make print labels for objects such as cans, cleaning supplies, and medications.

☑ Mark appliances at the most commonly used settings with a commercial labeling product that leaves bright and/or raised dots.

☑ Use everyday items, such as rubber bands, ribbons, electrical tape, or safety pins, that can either be felt or come in bright colors.

Safety First!

☑ Replace, move, or eliminate whenever possible objects that present a tripping hazard, such as throw rugs, worn carpeting, low tables, and clutter of all kinds.

☑ Take steps to improve visibility in areas where hazards cannot be eliminated, such as stairways and thresholds of doorways.

☑ Make sure cabinets and drawers are closed completely after every use and chairs are pushed under tables to avoid collisions.

☑ Keep all flammable items away from the stove.

☑ Follow manufacturers' safety precautions when using high-intensity or halogen lamps that produce intense heat, and never use a lightbulb that exceeds the recommended wattage of any light fixture.

that will help you to examine your own home environment. The next chapter takes a detailed look at the information you've collected from your assessment and discusses how to use it to make simple, low-cost changes in each room in your home and the everyday activities that take place there.

Lighting

Lighting is perhaps the most important factor to consider when you conduct a survey of your environment. Effective lighting can help you make the most of your vision. Since people usually need more light as they grow older, increasing the amount of light is one of the easiest ways to improve visibility in the home. There are a number of different types of light (see the box on "Types of Light in the Home"), so it is important not only to let in more light by opening up the curtains or blinds or getting an additional lamp, but also to match the type of light in an area to the activities that usually occur there.

As you walk around each room, look for areas that are inadequately or unevenly lit. Also look for places where *glare*—light reflected off shiny surfaces— makes it difficult to see. Glare can be caused by highly polished floors, shiny tabletops, mirrors, television screens and computer monitors, and chrome fixtures in bathrooms and kitchens. Some solutions for reducing glare in your home may include

● Switching to a nonglare floor wax

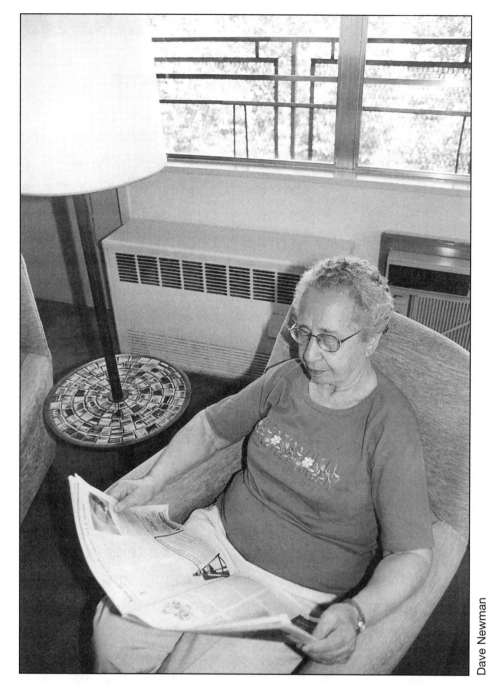

Dave Newman

Increase illumination by opening up the curtains to let in more light and bringing a lamp close to your task.

● Covering desktops or tabletops with tablecloths, runners, or place mats

● Repositioning mirrors and computer monitors

(Text continues on page 32)

Types of Light in the Home

When you think about ways to improve lighting around your home, consider the five different types of light that are currently available. Each has its own distinct characteristics and is appropriate for different activities. The Resource Guide at the back of this book lists some sources for different kinds of lighting, and many are available in independent living catalogs as well.

Sunlight/Natural Light

Although natural light is ideal for most everyday tasks, it is not always consistent throughout the day and tends to create dangerous shadowy areas and glare spots.

Incandescent Light

Since incandescent light is concentrated, it is best used in adjustable swing-arm lamps for intensive lighting for close activities, such as reading, writing, and sewing. It is not recommended for general room lighting, since, like sunlight, it tends to create shadowy areas and glare spots. Some points to remember about incandescent light:

☑ As the wattage increases, incandescent bulbs also produce more heat; therefore, they are usually not appropriate for prolonged close work, such as extended reading or detailed craft projects.

☑ Newer full-spectrum incandescent light bulbs (such as Chromalux bulbs) are closer to natural sunlight and produce a brighter, cleaner light for some individuals.

Fluorescent Light

Fluorescent lights are commonly seen in office buildings and schools; however, "warm" fluorescents can also be used in the home for general room lighting, since they light up a wider area than incandescents and do not create shadowy areas and glare spots.

☑ A new type of fluorescent light, called compact fluorescent bulbs (also called compact fluorescent lamps, or CFLs), fit into regular lamp sockets and provide illumination that is comparable to incandescent light, while producing less heat and using less energy.

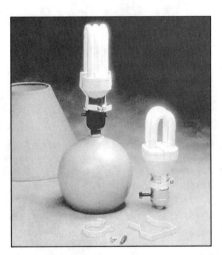 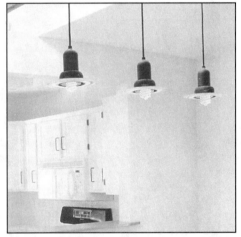

Phillips Lighting Company

Compact fluorescent bulbs fit into regular lamp sockets but have many of the advantages of fluorescent lights.

☑ Some fluorescent ceiling fixtures can be modified to minimize glare by replacing or retrofitting the louvers or "grills" that cover the fluorescent tubes.

Combination Light

A combination light, made up of both incandescent and fluorescent bulbs, is usually the most useful and comfortable light for most everyday activities. The combination of incandescent and fluorescent creates a type of light that is closest to natural sunlight.

☑ It is possible to combine fluorescent and incandescent lighting in the same fixture. Some adjustable swing-arm lamps contain a fluorescent "ring" that surrounds an incandescent lightbulb.

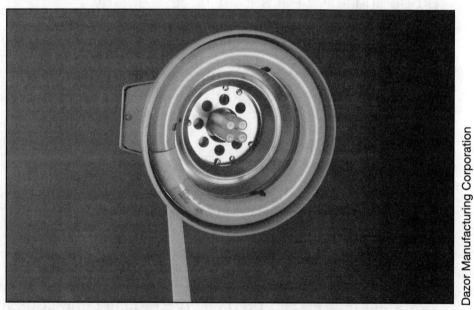

Dazor Manufacturing Corporation

Combining fluorescent and incandescent bulbs creates light that is closest to natural sunlight.

☑ Throughout your home, try to combine fluorescent and incandescent lighting whenever possible. Use fluorescents or CFLs for general room lighting, supplemented with incandescent bulbs in adjustable swing-arm desk and floor lamps.

Halogen Light

Some people prefer halogen light because it is brighter, "whiter," more concentrated, and more energy-efficient than incandescent light. It is used in lamps, track lighting, and recessed ceiling fixtures, and is also available in adjustable swing-arm lamps.

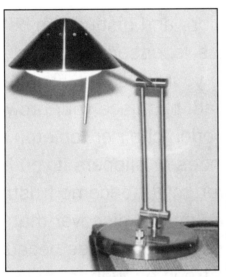
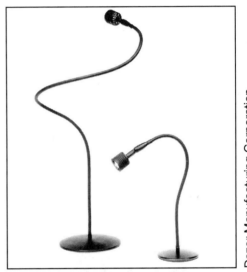

Dave Newman

Dazor Manufacturing Corporation

Halogen lights come in a variety of sizes and shapes. The light is very bright, but because it produces intense heat, it is not recommended for prolonged close work.

☑ Halogen light is hotter, more focused, and requires a shield; thus, it is not recommended for prolonged close work, such as reading, knitting, sewing, or crafts.

☑ Halogen light produces intense heat and can cause fire and severe burns and personal injury if used incorrectly. Always follow the manufacturer's safety precautions when using halogen lighting fixtures.

● Covering windows in bathrooms and kitchens with shades, miniblinds, or curtains

Improving the lighting in your home will not only make it easier to carry out all your everyday activities, but can also help you to see where you are walking and thus make your home safer.

Color and Contrast

The ability to perceive colors and distinguish between different color tones tends to lessen over time. You might occasionally "lose" your keys if you put them down on a floral bedspread, misplace your brown wallet if you leave it on a wooden chair or tabletop, or lose track of your dark shoes or slippers if you leave them on a dark carpet. You might become frustrated searching for these items, only to discover that they're "under your nose" but are difficult to see because the contrast or color wasn't strong enough to make them stand out. Enhancing the contrast between objects and their background and using strong, bright colors are among the simplest and most effective modifications you can make in your home to help you see and locate objects more easily.

When you walk through your home and examine your surroundings, look for places where lack of contrast makes objects difficult to see. Then try to think of ways that you can use color and contrast in different rooms to make you feel confident, secure, and safe. For example:

● Doorway thresholds are sometimes hard to see, and it may be difficult to judge their height correctly.

Painting each threshold in a bright solid color—red, orange, or yellow—sometimes helps. Although these colors may not match the surrounding furniture, they are usually much more visible than pastel colors and can prevent you from tripping or stumbling when you move from room to room.

● Color can help in the kitchen or bathroom, too. A strip of bright paint or striped warning tape along the edges of cabinet doors or drawers makes it easier to notice if they have been left open.

● Color-coding household files, documents, and forms by using a different color for each subject or category can make it easier to find the papers you need. Try Post-It notes in fluorescent colors, brightly colored stickers or paper clips, or brightly colored fluorescent markers.

● Color and contrast in table settings can prevent accidents and spills at the dinner table. White or light-colored plates against a dark tablecloth or place mats will usually provide the strongest contrast and make your dishes much easier to see. Avoid using clear glass cups and dishes because they are usually difficult to see.

● Try to place dark objects against lighter backgrounds, or vice versa. For example, a dark brown chair stands out best against white or cream-colored walls. If you can't make your furniture more visible by contrasting it with the background, try draping a white hand towel over the seat or back of a dark chair instead.

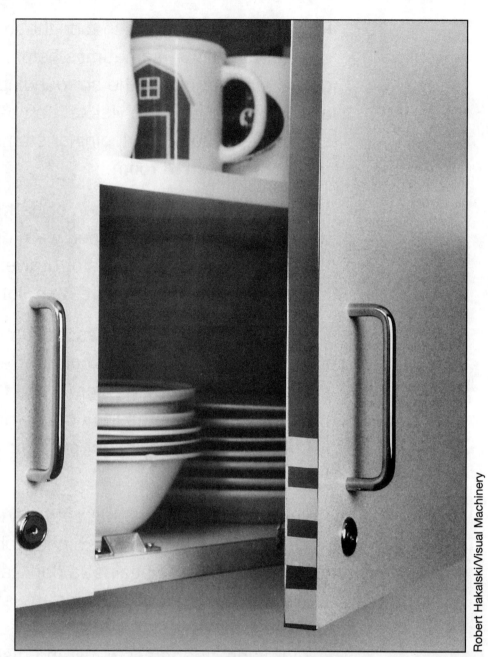

Robert Hakalski/Visual Machinery

A strip of bright, contrasting tape on the edge of a cabinet door makes it easier to see when it is left open.

Organization

How many times have you said to yourself, "One of these days, I'll *have* to get organized!" Applying principles of good organization, such as the ones listed in the

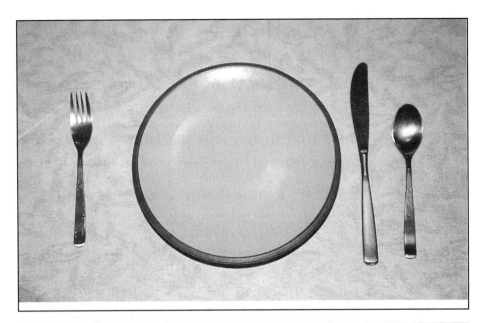

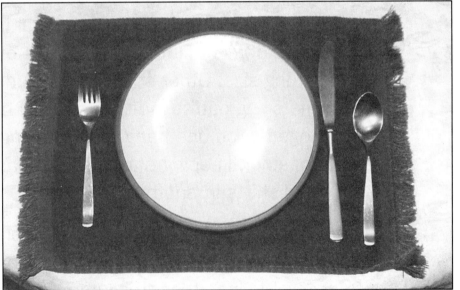

Ellen Bilofsky

A plate blends in with a tablecloth of the same color *(top)*, making it difficult to see. Placing a dark placemat in a contrasting color underneath the plate and silverware *(bottom)* improves visibility.

box earlier in this chapter, can help you find what you need when you need it. It can also help you avoid clutter that can get in your way or even cause accidents.

A good way to begin is to think about an organizational plan as you walk around your home. If you've lived in your home or apartment for a long time, you may have accumulated clutter that you always overlook, either because you've learned to live with it or because you feel secure with your home and belongings arranged in a particular way. Nevertheless, take a close look at potential trouble spots in your home, such as closets and cabinets, and try solutions such as these:

● Sometimes, a simple rearrangement of your closets may be all that is necessary to help you identify your outerwear, clothing, shoes, and accessories. If possible, separate your seasonal items and dispose of older clothing that is out of style or the wrong size. Other strategies include placing entire matching outfits (suit, shirt, belt, tie, and slacks) together on one hanger or grouping similar items together, keeping slacks in one part of the closet and shirts in another.

● In your drawers, use zipper-style plastic bags, ice cube trays, or egg cartons to separate and store jewelry and other small items.

● Look in bathroom cabinets and dispose of infrequently used or out-of-date prescription and nonprescription medications.

● In the kitchen, move frequently used appliances and supplies closer to the work area. Try arranging spices alphabetically. Group similar types of canned goods together, such as fruits, soups, or vegetables. Good organization skills can reduce the need for labeling and marking items.

● Develop regular schedules for activities you might otherwise overlook, such as when different areas of your home are likely to need cleaning. But also keep in mind that some tasks are best addressed immediately. For example, it takes much less effort to clean the stove top right after cooking than if you wait until food spills have had a chance to dry.

The next chapter provides additional suggestions for organizing different rooms in your home.

Texture and Touch

You may discover that you instinctively rely more and more on your sense of touch (or tactile sense) if your vision has decreased. Although it is not true that your sense of touch automatically becomes more sensitive to compensate for your vision loss, you can learn to pay closer attention to information that you receive through your hands and even feet. For example, instead of trying to identify a specific jacket or blazer through vision alone, you might also find it helpful to use your hands to search for distinguishing features, such as the texture of the fabric, buttons, and belts. Learning to use your tactile sense and becoming sensitive to the texture and "feel" of items in your home can help you feel more confident and in control of your surroundings. As you walk around your home, look for places where textures can give you information about objects or locations or where you can create tactile clues, such as the following:

- Attach an inexpensive textured decoration (even a piece of ribbon or a rubber band) to a bedroom doorknob to help you be certain that you're entering the right room.

- Use raised marking materials, such as a Hi-Marks 3-D Marker, Maxi-Marks, Bump Dots, or Spot 'n Line Pen, to make marks that you can feel (for sources of such materials, see Products for Independent Living in the Resource Guide at the back of this book). These materials can be used to label all kinds of items, from the settings on appliances, to medication bottles, to your apartment door. (See the section on Labels, Lettering, and Marking and Chapter 3 for more suggestions.)

- When you clean a tabletop or polish furniture, run your fingers lightly over the surface to determine its size, shape, and texture and to find any soiled areas that may need special treatment.

- When you pour cold liquids, such as milk, juice, or soda, use your fingers to feel the temperature change on the side of your glass or cup as the liquid rises.

- Your feet can give you valuable information, too. A carpeted floor that contrasts with the wooden floor in a hallway can help you to be sure that you are in a specific area in your home. (Try to eliminate scatter rugs whenever possible, however, since they may cause you to trip and possibly fall.)

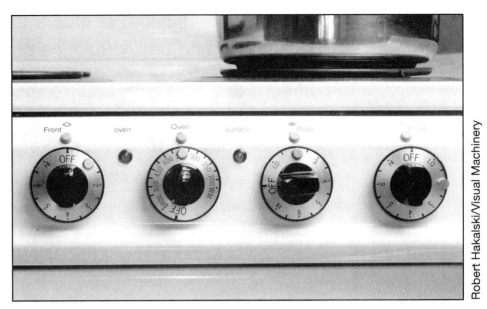

Robert Hakalski/Visual Machinery

These prepackaged raised marking dots with adhesive backs allow the user to feel when the stove dial is pointing to the right setting. Their bright red color adds a visual cue.

Sound

Just as you can use your sense of touch to obtain information, you can learn to pay more attention to sounds in the environment and rely on your sense of hearing to give you more information about your surroundings. For example:

● In the kitchen, you can use sounds to tell the difference between canned goods that may have the same size, shape, and weight; for example, when shaken, a can of fruit cocktail sounds different from a can of tomato paste.

● When you pour cold liquids, such as milk, juice, or soda, listen for the change in the sound to let you know when the liquid first enters the container, rises higher, and finally reaches the top.

In addition, technology related to the sense of hearing has been used to develop a number of reasonably priced products that can make your everyday life much easier. These so-called talking devices, such as microwaves, watches, clocks, scales, and calculators, can help you remain independent and safe when performing all types of everyday activities. For example:

- Electronic liquid-level indicators can help you pour hot and cold liquids by making a noise (and also vibrating) when the liquid in a glass or cup is a certain distance from the top rim.

- Cassette recorders and talking digital organizers can record and play back telephone numbers, addresses, memos, and appointments.

- Audio talk labels can identify clothing, food items, and medications. These labels consist of a blank card, about the size of an index card or credit card, that contains a magnetic recording strip or bar code. The card feeds into a small recording device while you speak a short description of the item that you wish to identify. The card can be attached to a medication bottle or other item with a rubber band. To identify the product, the card is run back through the machine to hear the spoken description.

Most of these products can be found in catalogs that specialize in products that promote independent living

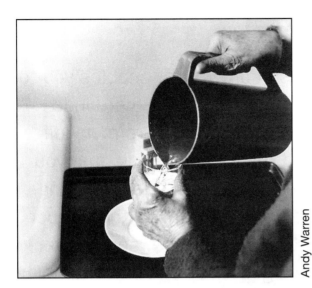
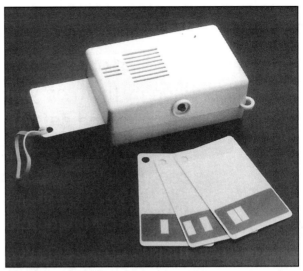

Andy Warren

Robert Hakalski/Visual Machinery

Technology can help us make use of the sense of hearing to get information about the environment. *(Left)* An electronic liquid level indicator (ELLI) hooks over the rim of a container and beeps when the liquid inside the container reaches the prongs—about an inch from the top. *(Right)* A form of labeling known as audio talk labels uses a small device to record brief descriptions of items on cards that contain a magnetic strip. The cards can be attached to the items with an elastic band. They are inserted back in the recorder so the descriptions can be played.

for people with vision loss or other disabilities. (A sample listing of these catalogs appears under Products for Independent Living in the Resource Guide at the back of this book.)

Make sure that you can hear the signal or "voice" from a device clearly before you purchase any of these items. Also, be aware that some everyday household noises (the dishwasher, television, or washing machine) can interfere with your hearing the sound from these devices. Try to locate and reduce background noise whenever possible.

Labels, Lettering, and Marking

Labeling or marking items in a way that enables you to identify them on your own can make you more independent and safer in your home. There are many different types of labels and marking materials that you can use to identify medications, food items, clothing, and cleaning products, as well as to mark the temperature settings on your stove, microwave, and toaster oven. Sometimes a labeling method can be as simple as placing a rubber band around a can of corn to distinguish it from a can of green beans or marking the lid of your blood pressure medication with a dot of fabric or craft paint. (If you label medications, however, be sure that you do not cover the print on the prescription portion of the label, since a friend or family member may need to read it in case of an emergency.)

Most of the following labeling methods use simple, low-cost materials and can reduce your need to ask for assistance with many everyday tasks, such as matching outfits, preparing meals, and grocery shopping:

■ Use a black wide-tip marker, a laundry marker, or a felt-tip pen to write in large, bold letters on plain white 3 x 5-inch index cards. Use these labels to differentiate household supplies that may be stored in similar spray containers, such as window cleaners, bathroom cleaners, and all-purpose cleaners. Attach each card to the appropriate container with a rubber band. As the containers become empty, you can remove the labels and take them to the store as a shopping list. Reattach the labels in the grocery store while the items are still in your shopping cart.

● Other types of everyday labeling materials include brightly colored plastic or electrical tape, safety pins, pipe cleaners, Velcro, fabric or craft paint, velour pads or furniture protectors, and iron-on patches.

● As mentioned earlier, there are also many special marking and labeling products such as Hi-Marks 3-D Marker or Spot 'n Line Pen that are available from catalogs specializing in products for people with visual impairments or other disabilities (see the Resource Guide).

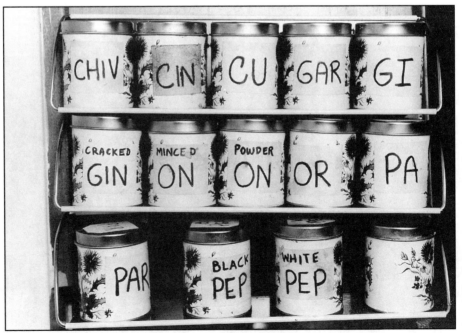

Simple, hand-written large-print labels attached with rubber bands identify these spices. Arranging the containers in alphabetical order also makes them easier to find.

■ Even if you do not read braille, you can use this system of raised dots to make useful tactile labels. A number of commercial products available for

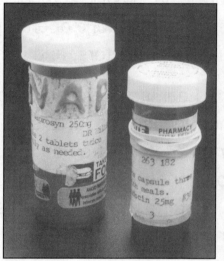

1

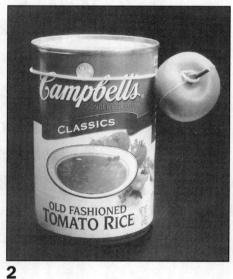

2

Robert Hakalski/Visual Machinery

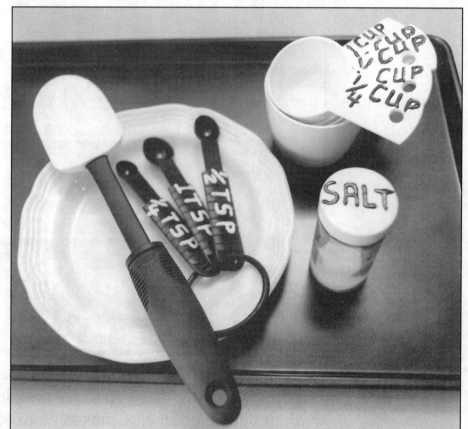

3

Andy Warren

marking and labeling in braille—such as aluminum clothing tags, braille labeling guns, magnetic labeling tape, and money braillers—are available from independent living products catalogs (see the Resource Guide).

Safety

Friends and family members often worry about the safety of an individual who has lost some vision. By following commonsense precautions, however, you can eliminate most safety hazards and prevent accidents. When you walk through your home, checking your surroundings and looking for problem areas, be sure to consider the following safety principles:

● Avoid long sleeves or loose-fitting clothing when you are cooking, and never reach across the stove top while you are wearing long or loose sleeves.

There are many methods of labeling using both specialized products and everyday household items: **(1)** The medicine container on the top left is labeled in large print using a commercial raised-marking substance, whereas the container on the right is identified simply with a rubber band. **(2)** A can of tomato rice soup is identified with a Loebel, a type of plastic food label that comes in the shape of various fruits and vegetables. **(3)** Various kitchen items are labeled with a raised-marking substance that takes advantage of contrast, large-print, and a tactile surface. Note also how the contrast of the items against the white plate and black tray increases the visibility of the items.

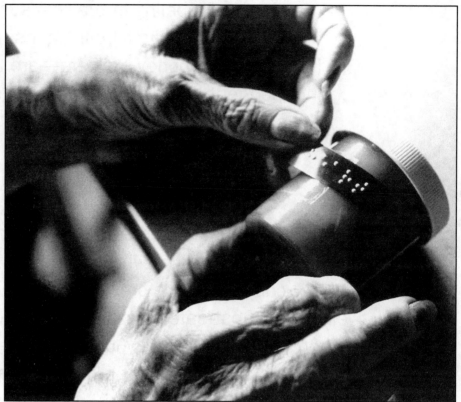

Braille dots on labeling tape make an excellent label that can be distinguished by touch, even if you don't read braille.

● Remove all flammable and combustible items from stove and counter tops, as well as from any storage area above the stove.

● Select a fire extinguisher that you can operate independently. Store it between the cooking area and the exit from the room.

● Periodically check that all electrical cords are in good condition, and replace any that are frayed or cracked.

● If any outlets or switches are unusually warm to the touch, have an electrician check the wiring as soon as possible, since this may indicate that the wiring is faulty.

● Move all extension and appliance cords away from the sink or range areas.

● Place at least one smoke detector on every floor of your home. Check and replace the batteries according to the manufacturer's instructions. A good rule of thumb is to replace batteries every spring and fall when you adjust your clocks.

● Position handles of pots and pans so they do not extend over the edge of the stove or over another burner.

● Unplug electrical appliances when not in use.

● Close cabinet doors and drawers immediately after use.

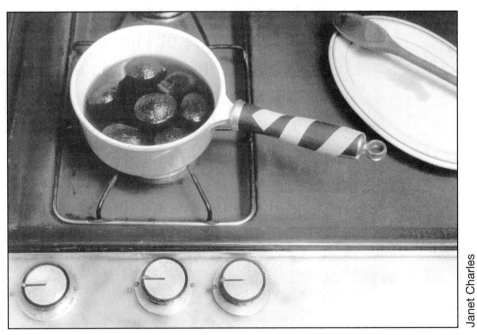

The handle of this pot is safely turned so it does not extend over the edge of the stove. Note also the contrasting tape wrapped around the handle and the contrast of the dark liquid with the light pot.

Getting Help in Assessing the Environment

The environmental elements and principles outlined in this chapter provide useful guidelines that enable older people with impaired vision to function independently and safely at home. Assistance in surveying your home is also available from people who are trained to do just that. *Rehabilitation teachers* are professionals in the field of vision rehabilitation who work with adults who are visually impaired to make environmental modifications within their homes and places of work. They also teach adaptive techniques for independent living. A rehabilitation teacher who provides independent living skills training in the older person's home can also assess the environment for safety and ease of functioning. Other professionals, called *orientation and mobility specialists,* who teach different methods of indoor and outdoor travel, also can help you make environmental modifications. (See "Where to Find Help" in Chapter 1 for information about how to find agencies that specialize in vision rehabilitation.)

The next chapter shows you how to apply the assessment guidelines discussed here. It examines each room and suggests specific solutions that you can implement on your own in your home and everyday activities.

HOME SURVEY CHECKLIST

Date: _____   Time: _____ A.M./P.M. (Circle one)

Room or area: _____

1. Lighting

What type of light is in this room or area? (Check all that apply.)

☐ Daylight/natural light ☐ Combination

☐ Incandescent ☐ Halogen

☐ Fluorescent

What type of lighting fixtures are in this room or area? (Check all that apply.)

☐ Ceiling lights

☐ Table lamps

☐ Light fixture or lamp with a dimmer switch

☐ Natural light/windows

☐ Other (describe) _____

☐ No light in this area

Describe the levels of light in this area:

☐ Too bright ☐ Uneven (alternating bright and dark areas)

☐ Too dim/dark ☐ Adequate

Recommendations for change:

_____

_____

_____

_____

_____

_____

2. *Glare*

Are there shiny surfaces in this room or area? (Check all that apply.)

- ☐ Polished floors
- ☐ Mirrors
- ☐ Tabletops
- ☐ Computer monitor or television screen
- ☐ Shiny or glossy paint or wallpaper
- ☐ Chrome fixtures in the sink area
- ☐ Other (describe)

_____

_____

_____

Are there windows in this area?

- ☐ Covered with adjustable drapes, shades, blinds
- ☐ Uncovered
- ☐ Skylights
- ☐ Other (describe) _____

Recommendations for change:

_____

_____

_____

_____

_____

_____

3. *Color and Contrast*

What color are the walls?
- ☐ White
- ☐ Pastel
- ☐ Dark
- ☐ Patterned or striped wall covering

What color is the floor covering?
- ☐ White
- ☐ Pastel
- ☐ Dark
- ☐ Patterned or striped

What color is the furniture?
- ☐ White
- ☐ Pastel
- ☐ Dark
- ☐ Patterned or striped

Is there sufficient contrast . . .
- ☐ Yes ☐ No between the door frame, door, and walls?
- ☐ Yes ☐ No between the walls and floor?
- ☐ Yes ☐ No between furniture and the walls?
- ☐ Yes ☐ No between handrails and the walls?
- ☐ Yes ☐ No between the print and the background?

Recommendations for change:

_____

_____

_____

_____

_____

_____

4. *Organization*

Do you notice any "cluttered" areas that need reorganization?

☐ Yes ☐ No Closets
☐ Yes ☐ No Cupboards
☐ Yes ☐ No Drawers
☐ Yes ☐ No Cabinets
☐ Yes ☐ No Tabletops/desktops
☐ Yes ☐ No On steps/stairs

Recommendations for change:

_____

_____

_____

_____

5. *Safety Hazards*

☐ Yes ☐ No Are there any flammable items near heat sources?
☐ Yes ☐ No Are all electrical cords in good condition?
☐ Yes ☐ No Are any outlets or switches warm to the touch?
☐ Yes ☐ No Are all smoke alarms in working order?

☐ Yes   ☐ No   Is there a fire extinguisher in place (if appropriate)?

☐ Yes   ☐ No   Other safety hazards (describe) _____

_____

Recommendations for change:

_____

_____

_____

_____

_____

6. Can you add texture cues in this area?

Recommendations for change:

_____

_____

_____

_____

_____

7. Can you add sound cues in this area?

Recommendations for change:

_____

_____

_____

_____

_____

8. *Can you add* labels, lettering, *or* marking *in this area?*

Recommendations for change:

_____

_____

_____

_____

_____

Modifying Your Environment: Room by Room

The basic principles discussed in the previous chapter—avoiding clutter; using good organizational techniques; and making maximum use of contrast, color, and appropriate lighting—can be applied to every room in your home. When you consider possible changes or modifications for a specific area in your home or for your everyday activities, try to keep the following guidelines in mind:

- Involve your family members and friends and work together to find solutions for the problem areas you identify.

- If you mark or label an item in your home, such as your stove dials, microwave panel, or medication containers, make sure that everyone in your household can understand and use your marking system.

- Avoid covering up the numbers or words on your medication bottles with dots or other markings that will prevent others from reading your prescription information.

- Whenever possible, plan the changes you make so that you can maintain them independently and with a minimum of effort. For instance, if you use tape or paint to mark your steps or stairs, you should be able to repair or replace these markings on your own when they become worn.

- Pay special attention to safety precautions for the bathroom, the area next to the bed, the hallway, and steps and stairs because these are the most common places for falls.

There is no "one size fits all" solution that is right for everyone. No two people have the same type and degree of vision loss; the same lifestyle; the same kind of home; or the same needs, wants, and preferences. There are usually several ways to address a specific environmental situation or problem, and the suggestions that follow are simply examples to help you develop solutions that are best for you. Be creative, involve your family members and friends, and remember that most modifications can be simple, safe, practical, and inexpensive.

Adaptations for Every Room

A good way to begin is to think about overall changes or modifications that you can apply to every room in your home (see Chapter 2 for basic principles). Keep in mind that the ideas outlined here are only suggestions, and it's likely that you will discover many equally useful solutions that apply to your specific situation.

Lighting

▶▶ Use additional sources of light, such as adjustable swing-arm and gooseneck lamps, for activities that require brighter, more concentrated light.

▶▶ Use dimmer switches for room lighting and three-way bulbs in lamps to give you more flexibility as your lighting needs change throughout the day.

▶▶ Paint switch plates in solid, bright colors or outline them with fluorescent tape or paint to increase their visibility. Use glow-in-the-dark switches or a switch with a night light for nighttime use.

▶▶ Do not exceed the recommended wattage of any lighting fixture, since injury or even fire can result.

▶▶ Replace darker lamp shades with lighter-colored ones that allow the maximum amount of light to pass through.

Floor coverings

▶▶ Tack or tape down the corners and edges of rugs. Remove rugs and runners that tend to slide or apply double-faced adhesive carpet tape or rubber matting to the backs of all floor coverings.

▶▶ Pull up and replace worn and torn carpeting and linoleum. Check rugs or runners periodically to determine if the backing needs to be replaced.

▶▶ Cover bare and potentially slippery floors with textured runners or carpeting. Try to use carpeting with a short nap, if possible, since this surface can provide more stability when walking.

▶▶ Use solid-colored carpeting, linoleum, or tile, which may be less visually confusing than patterned or "checkerboard" floor coverings.

Thresholds and door sills

▶▶ To prevent tripping on thresholds or door sills, bevel or plane them down if possible so they are flush or no more than a quarter-inch height and paint them in bright solid colors.

▶▶ Paint doors, doorknobs, and door frames in bright solid colors to increase their visibility and enable you to locate doors and exits quickly in case of an emergency.

▶▶ Wear snug-fitting shoes or slippers with backs to prevent slips on any uneven areas of the floor.

Window coverings

▶▶ Use miniblinds or vertical shades to control direct sunlight; adjust them for different lighting conditions according to the weather and time of day.

You can also use them in combination with sheer or lace window coverings to match decor.

▶▶ Avoid hanging planters, mobiles, and other window decorations that can block sunlight and cause shadows.

After you apply these general principles to your home as a whole, go room by room to think about specific changes you might want to make, as well as the everyday tasks that you need to do within each room. Try to think about your lighting requirements before you begin to make other changes, since lighting is the most important change that you can make in every area of your home. In this chapter you will find two sets of suggestions for each room. The first set outlines ways to adapt the room and its contents, while the second set suggests alternative ways to perform the activities that are usually done in that part of the house. Again, these suggestions are only guidelines; use them to stimulate your own ideas and ingenuity in developing practical solutions.

Remember, too, that if you think you need additional help with any area discussed in this book, you can contact a local vision rehabilitation agency for information (see "Where to Find Help" in Chapter 1 or the sources of information and referrals listed in the Resource Guide at the back of this book). Finally, most of the adapted products mentioned in this chapter, unless otherwise specified, are available from independent living catalogs that specialize in products for people who are visually impaired or have other disabilities. See the Resource Guide at the end of this book for a sampling of such catalog companies.

Kitchen and Dining Area

It's likely that you spend a considerable amount of time in the kitchen and dining area of your home, since this is usually the center of activity in most households. When you think about changes you can make in this area, it's important to consider the range of safety issues that are associated with preparing meals, cooking, and using a variety of electrical appliances. By experimenting with simple changes in lighting, color, and contrast, you can make cooking and other kitchen activities safer.

Adaptations

▶▶ Attach lights to the underside of cabinets over work areas, below eye level and shielded to keep light out of your eyes. Try to use warm fluorescent or compact fluorescent bulbs whenever possible.

▶▶ Install adjustable swing-arm or gooseneck lamps near appliances that you use frequently or use a floor lamp on wheels that will allow you to move the light with you as you move around the kitchen area.

▶▶ Remove any towels that are hanging on the oven handle. If any towels are located close to a burner, change the location of the towel rack.

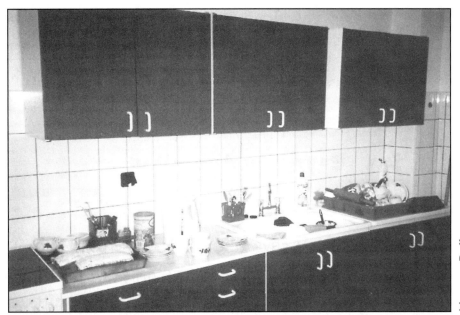

Cabinet doors painted in a dark color with contrasting handles stand out against a kitchen's white walls.

▶▶ Make it a habit to close cupboard and cabinet doors as soon as you remove or replace an item.

▶▶ Paint cabinet doors in a solid bright color to make them stand out against the walls and counters. Replace cabinet hardware with brightly colored contrasting handles.

▶▶ Learn to listen or feel for clicks as you turn knobs to different stove and oven settings. Ask if the manufacturer will supply new dials or knobs if yours are worn or covered with built-up cooking grime.

▶▶ Check with the manufacturer of your appliances to see if it is possible to obtain braille overlays for dials. Even if you don't know braille, raised dots can help you to identify settings by touch.

‣ Mark your stove dials or microwave panel with dots of glue or with specialized commercial products, such as Hi-Marks 3-D Marker, Maxi-Marks, Bump Dots, or Spot 'n Line Pen, usually found in specialty catalogs.

 Everyday Activities

Cooking

‣ Always use flame-retardant elbow-length oven mitts when removing hot pans from the stove or oven. Make sure the oven mitts are dry, since water allows heat to come through.

‣ Turn off the oven and stove dials *before* you remove pots and pans. Stand off to the side when you open the oven door, not directly in front of it.

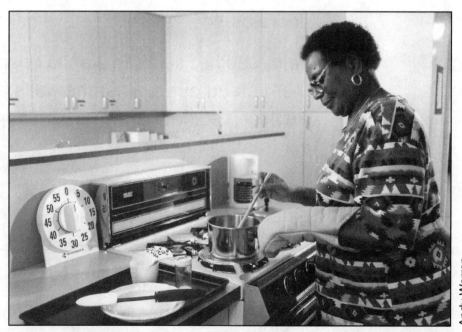

This cook makes use of several safety products, including long oven mitts and a flame tamer to protect against burns. Note the kitchen timer with large numerals at left.

▶▶ Use large-print recipes and cookbooks (available from some specialty catalogs) and place them in a cookbook holder or on a reading stand while you work.

▶▶ Use a kitchen timer with large-print or tactile markings.

▶▶ To hold a pot steady while moving it, place it in a broiler pan, cake pan, or tray before you attempt to carry it to the work area.

▶▶ Wrap plastic tape of a contrasting color around pot handles to make them more visible.

▶▶ Keep one dark and one light cutting board on hand. Use the dark one to contrast with light-colored foods, such as potatoes, and use the light one for slicing colored foods, such as tomatoes and green peppers. Similarly, use dark-colored bowls for mixing flour and lighter cake mixes, and use a white or light-colored bowl for darker ingredients.

▶▶ Attach light and dark sheets of contact paper to the counter and to a spot on the wall near your food preparation area. Hold up dark ingredients against light-colored sheets and light ingredients against dark.

▶▶ To keep track of how much salt you're adding to a recipe, pour it into your hand first, and then feel when you have the specified amount. This technique also works for most herbs and spices.

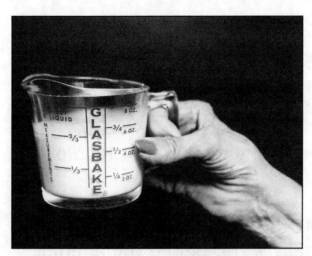 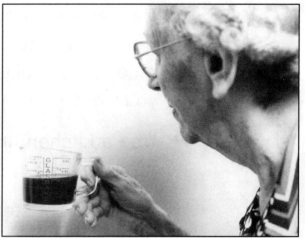

Janet Charles

Contrast helps in the kitchen. Light liquids contrast well with a dark piece of paper or shelving paper glued to the wall *(left);* **dark liquids show up against a light wall** *(right).*

▶▶ Organize and label canned and boxed foods with any of the methods described in Chapter 2.

▶▶ Hang your most frequently used pots and pans on a pegboard within easy reach.

▶▶ Store knives in a knife holder or with protective covers over the blades.

▶▶ When pouring *cold* liquids only, place your index finger at the rim of the cup, listen for sound changes as the container fills, and feel the temperature change on the side of the glass or cup.

▶▶ You can also use an electronic liquid-level indicator, as described in Chapter 2, to help you pour hot liquids more safely. A Hot Shot hot water dispenser also heats and serves one cup of hot water at a time.

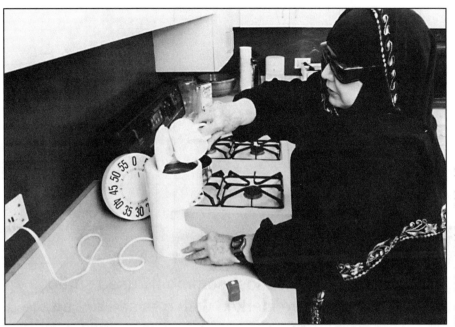

This Hot Shot hot water dispenser boils a single cup of water and dispenses it into a mug at the push of a button to make one cup of tea, instant coffee, hot chocolate, or soup. Note the electronic liquid-level indicator on the plate at front.

Laundry

▶▶ If you have laundry facilities in your home, install adjustable swing-arm lighting over the washing machine and dryer and use a handheld magnifier to read the controls.

▶▶ Mark frequently used settings with a Hi-Marks 3-D Marker, Maxi-Marks, Bump Dots, or Spot 'n Line Pen or check to see if the manufacturer supplies braille overlays.

▶▶ If you are purchasing a new washing machine, look for one that has a minimum of complicated settings and features easy-to-use dials.

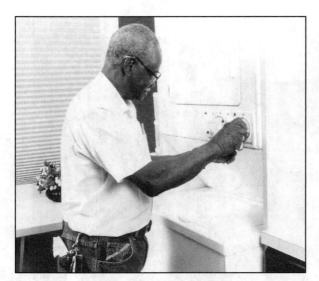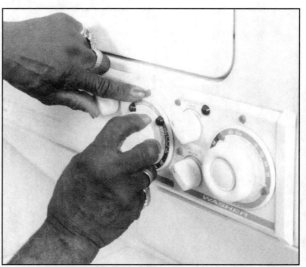

Robert Hakalski/Visual Machinery

The most commonly used settings on these dryer dials are marked with a raised dot so the user can feel when the dials point to the correct setting.

▶▶ To help with ironing, install adjustable swing-arm lighting over the work area; mark frequently used heat settings with a Hi-Marks 3-D Marker, Maxi-Marks, Bump Dots, or Spot 'n Line Pen; and use a solid, nonpatterned ironing board cover.

▶▶ When reaching for the iron, locate the cord first and then follow it to the handle.

▶▶ Use a funnel to pour water into a steam iron.

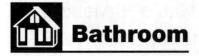 Bathroom

The bathroom requires special attention because glare from chrome fixtures and glossy tile can combine with slippery tub and floor surfaces to create hazardous conditions that can lead to falls. Lighting, safety issues, and sources of glare are important factors to consider in this room.

Adaptations

▶▶ Experiment with different lightbulbs in your light fixtures: try full-spectrum or compact fluorescent bulbs or increase the wattage of the bulbs you are currently using (see Chapter 2 for details). Remember not to exceed the recommended wattage of any lighting fixture.

▶▶ Install adjustable swing-arm lamps wherever you need additional lighting for combing your hair or applying makeup. Gather up the excess electrical cord with an automatic windup reel or even a rubber band.

▶▶ Replace any accent or area rugs with a floor mat with nonskid backing or wall-to-wall carpeting in a color that contrasts with the walls and fixtures.

▶▶ When purchasing towels, washcloths, and bath mats, choose solid colors that contrast with the bathtub, floor, and wall tile.

▶▶ For additional safety and security, install grab bars by the toilet and in the shower and tub area. Wrapping them with brightly colored contrasting tape makes them highly visible in case you need to reach for them quickly. Don't use the soap dish or toilet paper holder instead of a grab bar because you can pull it out of the wall if you lean on it too heavily.

▶▶ Replace a white toilet seat with a brightly colored one that contrasts with the walls and fixtures.

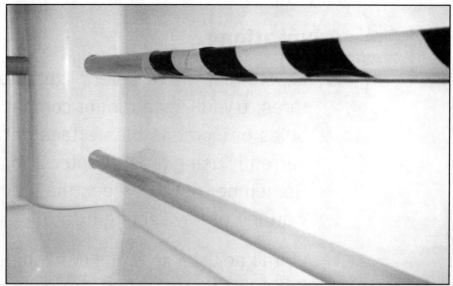

Maureen Duffy

A grab bar in the bathtub can be made highly visible by wrapping it with contrasting tape.

▶▶ Drape a contrasting bath mat over the edge of the tub to make it easier to see.

▶▶ Apply a strip of contrasting colored tape along the entire edge of the tub.

▶▶ Place a contrasting nonskid textured mat in the shower or tub to prevent falls and provide a cue for judging the depth of the bathtub when you step into it.

▶▶ Set the control on your hot water heater to a medium-range temperature to reduce the danger of scalding.

▶▶ Transfer soap, shampoo, and other bath products to brightly colored plastic bottles and containers that contrast with the tub and wall tile. Use a shower caddy to organize your bath products. A

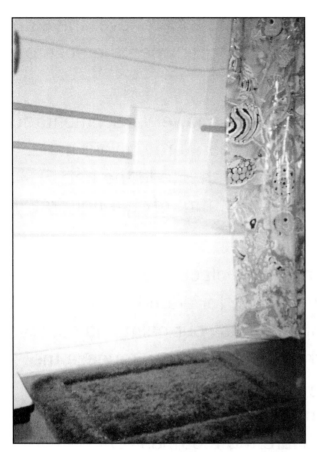 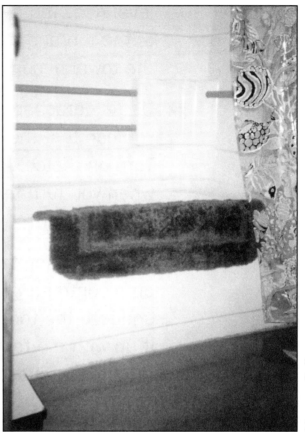

Hanging a contrasting bath mat over the edge of a white bathtub makes it easier to see the side of the tub.

rubber band around the shampoo bottle will distinguish it from the conditioner.

☀ Everyday Activities

Personal Hygiene and Grooming

▸▸ Use "soap-on-a-rope" to help you locate your soap more easily and prevent you from slipping on it or dropping it in the tub or shower.

▸▸ To fill the bathtub to the correct level, place a contrasting strip of tape at the correct depth or float a brightly colored toy in the water so you can see the level rise. You can also drape a towel over the side of the tub and turn off the water when the edge of the towel becomes wet.

▶▶ Use a detachable handheld shower attachment, so you can test the water temperature on your hand. Turn on the cold water first, then add the hot; when you turn the water off, turn off the hot first, then the cold.

▶▶ When applying toothpaste, place the toothbrush on a contrasting washcloth for added visibility; squeeze the toothpaste into your palm and scoop it up with the toothbrush bristles; or squeeze the toothpaste directly into your mouth from the dispenser. (The last method is recommended only if no other persons share the toothpaste.)

▶▶ Place your free hand over the top of the faucet to serve as a point of reference and to help you avoid hitting it or emptying your mouth over it when you are brushing your teeth.

▶▶ To monitor your weight, use a talking scale, available in speciality catalogs.

Identifying Medications

▶▶ Organize medications in alphabetical order.

▶▶ Separate medications by location: breakfast pills in the kitchen and nighttime pills in the bedroom.

▶▶ Ask your pharmacist to make a large-print label for each bottle.

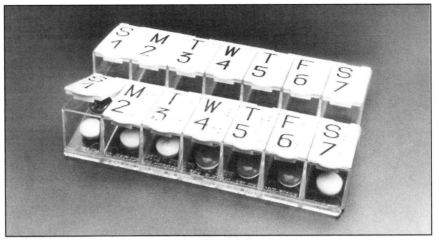

1

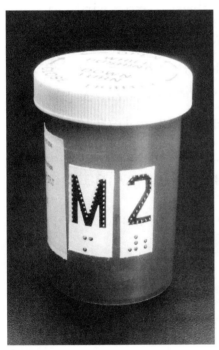

2

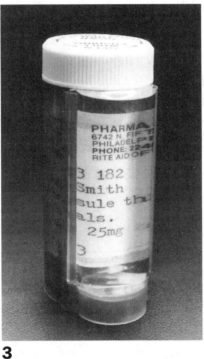

3

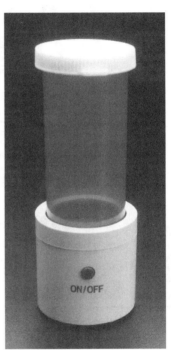

4

There are many ways to keep track of medication: **(1)** This pill box stores two weeks' worth of pills in compartments labeled for each day of the week in tactile large print and braille. **(2)** This medicine container is labeled with a combination of large print, tactile marking (raised dots along the letters), and braille. **(3)** Medicine containers fit into this special sleeve with a built-in magnifier that enlarges the label, **(4)** and a talking prescription label system uses a device to "read" out loud an electronic label on the medicine container.

▶▶ Store your pills in pill boxes that have separate compartments for each day of the week. These boxes can be found in some drug stores as well as in specialty catalogs.

▶▶ Label your medications with any of the methods described in Chapter 2.

▶▶ Use rubber bands to differentiate medications that are stored in similar containers.

▶▶ Ask your pharmacist about talking prescription labels. This identification system produces a special electronic "label" for each medicine container to identify its contents. When the container is placed in a special base that you keep in your home, the device will "read" the label out loud. (See the Resource Guide for more information.)

▶▶ Dispose of old or outdated medications promptly.

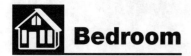 **Bedroom**

One important consideration in the bedroom is safety, since a great number of falls occur in the area next to the bed. For example, if you have to get up in the middle of the night, you may find that your bedside light is either too bright or too dim when you awaken, or you may not be able to find your eyeglasses in the darkness. Changing the type of lamps or room lighting in your bedroom, combined with some commonsense safety precautions, can provide a number of effective solutions. Other concerns in the bedroom involve identifying and matching your clothing and keeping clothing in good repair.

 ## Adaptations

▶▶ Replace your wall switch with a dimmer switch and use an extension cord and a dimmer switch for your bedside lamp. Make sure that you gather up the excess electrical cord with an automatic windup reel or rubber band.

▶▶ Install adjustable swing-arm or gooseneck lamps wherever you need additional lighting for reading, or identifying your clothing or medication. In your closets, install battery-operated lights that can be mounted on the wall.

▶▶ Get a bedside lamp that you can activate by clapping your hands or by simply touching the base.

▶▶ Keep a night light on throughout the night. Install one in your bedroom, one in your bathroom, and one in the hallway, if needed.

▶▶ Place a small lamp just inside the door of your bedroom and switch it on to help you find your bedside light.

▶▶ Remove any accent or area rugs that you can't tape down or otherwise secure.

▶▶ Attach a bed caddy to the side of your bed to hold smaller items, such as eyeglasses, tissues, and medication containers.

▶▶ If possible, remove the footboard of your bed, since you can be injured if you fall against it. For some individuals, however, the footboard can be useful as a guide or support. If you can't remove the footboard, make up the bed with a thick blanket or quilt over the sharp corners of the footboard.

▶▶ Make it a habit to close closet doors or dresser drawers immediately after you use them.

▶▶ Always put your shoes and slippers away (in your closet or under your bed) as soon as you remove them.

 Everyday Activities

Organizing Clothing

▶▶ Organize and label your clothing, accessories, and shoes with any of the methods described in Chapter 2.

▶▶ To label clothing items, try any of the following items: small brass "no rust" laundry pins, iron-on patches in various sizes and shapes, buttons, or a variety of commercial marking systems sold in independent living catalogs.

▶▶ Use color-coded storage boxes for your clothing and accessories; for example, use brown for winter clothing; red for summer clothing; and white for hats, gloves, and scarves. You can also label each storage box with any of the methods described in Chapter 2.

▶▶ Use plastic clips, known as "sock locks" or "sock tuckers," to keep matching socks together in the washer and dryer and in the drawer. These clips can be found commercially as well as in specialty catalogs.

▶▶ If it is difficult to reach items on the top shelf of your closet, either reorganize and store them in your drawers or use a "reacher" or "grabber" to bring them closer for identification. These long, scissor-like devices with rubber tips for gripping objects are sold both commercially and in specialty catalogs.

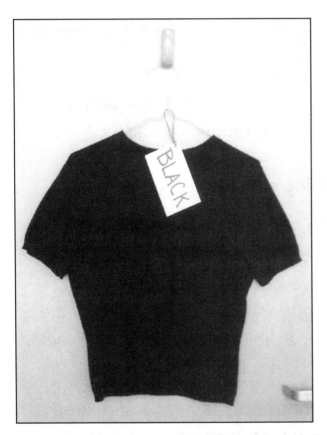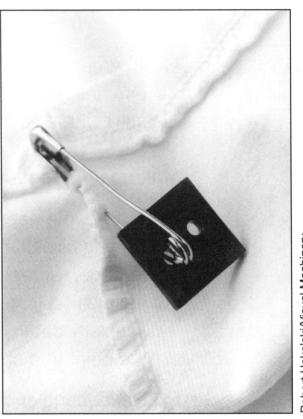

A variety of both homemade and commercial systems exist to label clothing for easy identification, among them, large-print labels that can be attached to a hanger *(left)*. Another system uses durable plastic tags in different shapes that can be pinned to garments *(right)*.

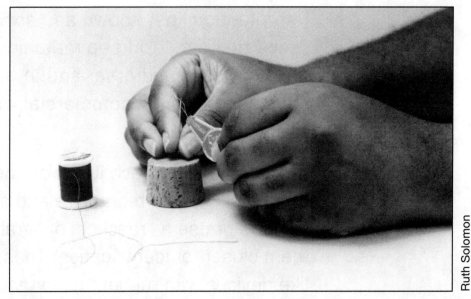

Ruth Solomon

Stabilizing a needle in a cork or a bar of soap while using a wire loop threader makes the task of threading a needle much simpler.

▶▶ To group all parts of a matching outfit together, use hangers that allow you to combine pants or a skirt with a coordinating blouse or shirt.

Making simple clothing repairs

▶▶ To thread a needle, install adjustable swing-arm lighting over the work area and use a wire loop threader, spread-eye needles, or self-threading needles (sold in both sewing notions stores and specialty catalogs). Stabilize the needle by placing the point in a cork or a bar of soap.

▶▶ Place fabric on a contrasting surface and keep a magnet nearby to pick up pins and needles. Use a wrist pin cushion in addition to a regular one.

▶▶ Keep several pre-threaded needles on hand for emergency repairs.

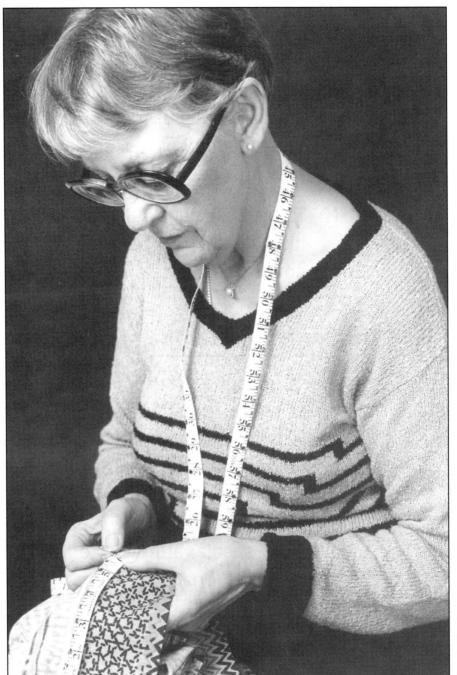

Janet Charles

This tape measure has holes at regular intervals that can be felt as well as seen. You can count the holes to measure the fabric, and pins can be inserted in the holes to mark a spot. The large heads on the straight pins being used here make them easier to see.

▶▶ Use an adapted tape measure that has holes to indicate 1" and ½" intervals.

▶▶ When purchasing thread, ask the clerk to make sure the ends of the thread on new spools are loose instead of tucked under or in a slot where they may be hard to find.

▶▶ To avoid sticking yourself on fallen pins or needles, do not sew barefoot or when wearing thin socks or slippers.

 # Study or Home Office

Everyone has a place where he or she reads mail, writes letters, makes telephone calls, pays bills, and, perhaps, uses a computer, even if it is a simple alcove or the kitchen table. These activities are crucial to maintaining your household and finances independently. Regardless of where you do these kinds of activities, pay special attention to lighting, color, contrast, and organization in this area.

 ## Adaptations

▶▶ Install adjustable swing-arm and gooseneck lamps in areas where you will be reading, writing, and paying bills or use a floor lamp on wheels that will allow you to move the light with you as you move around your work area.

▶▶ Place a strip of fluorescent warning tape on the edges of desk and file cabinet drawers to alert you when they are open and to avoid potential accidents.

▶▶ Always close drawers immediately after using them; also, push chairs under tables and return all materials to their original location whenever you complete a task.

▶▶ Color-code your household files, documents, and forms with fluorescent Post-It notes, colored stickers or paper clips, or brightly colored fluorescent markers.

▶▶ If your desk or writing surface is shiny or glossy, cover it with a cloth or desk pad to minimize glare.

☀ Everyday Activities

▶▶ To write a letter or shopping list, place the sheet of paper on a contrasting surface, such as a clipboard or darker piece of paper, to minimize glare and give you a better idea of the size and shape of the writing area.

▶▶ If you need more contrast, use bold-line paper with a black felt-tip marker, such as a Flair or 20/20 pen. This will help you to see where you are writing, and will also help you to stay on the lines as you write.

▶▶ When you need to sign documents, insurance forms, or greeting cards, use a signature guide—a plastic, cardboard, or metal template that will out-

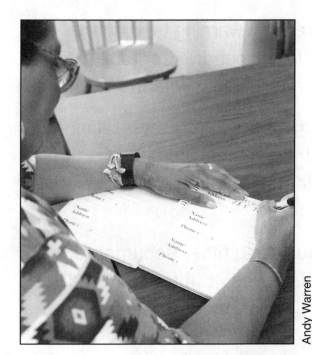

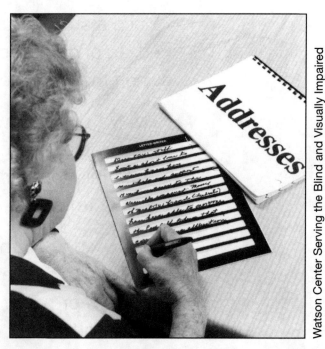

Bold-line pages, as in this large-print address book, and a black felt-tip marker *(left),* are effective tools for easier writing. A high-contrast writing guide *(right)* allows you to both feel and see where the lines are as you write.

line the space where your signature belongs. Similar templates are also available to help you write letters, address envelopes, and fill out checks. (See the Resource Guide for more information.)

▶▶ To maintain your check deposit register, use bold-line paper with a black felt-tip marker. You may also wish to ask if your bank will provide large-print checks and deposit registers.

▶▶ A closed-circuit television is a reading device that will enlarge the print on a page or a document and project it onto a large screen or monitor. Your low vision specialist can tell you more about this

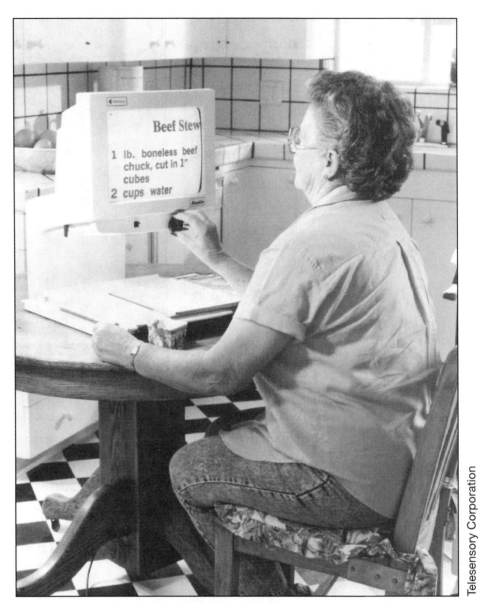

Telesensory Corporation

A closed-circuit television system (CCTV) can enlarge the print on all kinds of reading material for many people with low vision.

device and whether it is appropriate for your needs and specific eye condition.

▶▶ Use telephones with large-print push buttons or large-print dial overlays. Make sure that the numbers are large enough to see and are printed in a

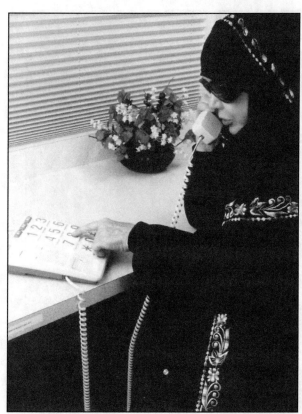 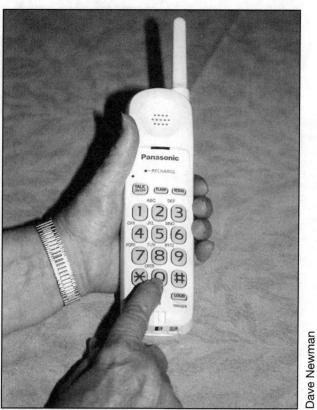

Dave Newman

Telephones with high-contrast, large-print numbers *(left)* make dialing easier. A cordless telephone with large numbers *(right)* can provide additional flexibility.

color that provides good contrast with the color of the telephone.

▶▶ Using a cordless telephone with high-contrast, large-print numbers will allow you to move the dial as close as you need to see the numbers clearly. Sometimes this type of telephone can provide more flexibility than a unit that is attached to the wall or placed on a desktop.

▶▶ Many telephones have features that enable you to program frequently dialed numbers into your keypad. To dial a number, it is only necessary to push two buttons, instead of seven or even ten numbers.

▶▶ Persons who are visually impaired are eligible for free operator-assistance programs. These plans allow you to call directory assistance and have a number dialed for you at no extra charge. Your local telephone company can supply you with information.

▶▶ If you are having difficulty reading your computer screen, try repositioning the monitor to minimize glare on the screen, adjusting the size and font of the type that is displayed, or investing in a larger monitor. You can also buy software that will increase the size of the text on your screen. (Some independent living catalogs carry such software.)

▶▶ To make it easier to find the correct keys on the computer keyboard, mark the home-row keys with one of the tactile marking materials described in Chapter 2, or use large-print adhesive-backed key covers (sold in independent living catalogs).

Living Room

Lighting is frequently a problem in living rooms, which may have either too much sunlight streaming in from uncovered windows or too little light because window treatments block useful daylight. In addition, living room furniture may have sharp edges, and low-lying coffee tables in particular can cause injuries and falls. Since many people use the living room for watching television and reading, as well as for conversation, it is important to combine an attractive and pleasing environment with recommended lighting and safety modifications.

Adaptations

▶▶ Replace darker lamp shades with lighter-colored ones and experiment with different lightbulbs in existing light fixtures. Try full-spectrum or compact fluorescent bulbs or change the wattage of the bulbs you are currently using (see Chapter 2 for more information). Install adjustable swing-arm or gooseneck lamps in areas where you will be reading books, newspapers, and magazines and experiment with the position of the light to determine what works best for you. Remember not to exceed the recommended wattage of any lighting fixture.

▶▶ Use a lamp with a "clap-on" feature or one that you can activate by simply touching the base.

▶▶ Tack down or use double-sided tape on all runners and area rugs. Tape down all edges of rugs that receive heavy foot traffic.

▶▶ Rearrange the furniture, if space permits, to keep low coffee tables or anything with sharp edges out of the path of travel. Use a bright towel or tablecloth to pad the edges and corners of furniture that cannot be moved.

▶▶ Also, think about rearranging your furniture to give you a place to pause if you need to adjust to changes in lighting levels between bright and dark areas, such as when you enter your living room from a dim hallway.

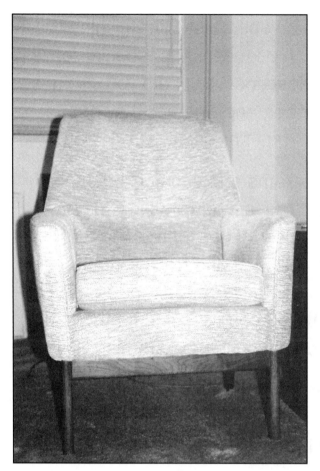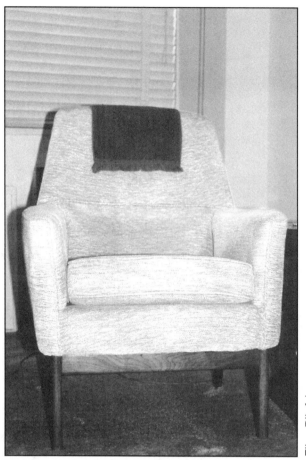

A brightly colored, contrasting towel draped over the back of a chair helps it stand out against the wall.

▸▸ Mark your favorite chair with a brightly colored cushion to help you locate it more easily or cover the chair with a solid, brightly colored slipcover or drape a towel over the back to make it stand out in contrast to the wall.

☼ Everyday Activities

▸▸ If you find it difficult to see the television picture, it may be helpful to place the television on a rolling cart so you can move it closer or change its position if there is glare on the screen.

▶▶ Consult your low vision specialist to determine if specific devices, such as magnifiers, special reading glasses, or small telescopes, will help you see the television or read better, and whether they are appropriate for your needs and specific eye condition.

▶▶ Some television programs and films on videotape are available in video-described versions; that is, they have explanations and descriptions of the visual elements inserted on the sound track without interfering with the sounds and dialogue that are part of the program. See the Resource Guide for more information on how to obtain such programming.

▶▶ Use a clipboard or reading stand to hold the pages of reading material closer to you to eliminate unnecessary bending and stretching.

▶▶ If reading regular print is difficult or impossible, even after following these suggestions, consider obtaining large-print books or recorded books on tape. Some large-print periodicals, such as the *New York Times* and *Reader's Digest,* are available through subscription. The Library of Congress Talking Book Program makes available a wide variety of Talking Books, along with a tape machine on which to play them. This service is free of charge to individuals who are blind or visually impaired through local or regional libraries for the blind. (See the Resource Guide for more sources of large-print reading materials and Talking Books.)

▶▶ Radio reading services that broadcast newspapers and other printed materials are provided by certain radio stations, which provide closed-circuit radio receivers and program listings to subscribers. (See the Resource Guide for more information.)

 ## Steps, Stairs, and Hallways

Because they are thought of as passages, not rooms, steps, stairs, and hallways are often ignored and frequently are poorly lit. The most compelling reason that most older adults give for moving from their homes can be summarized in one word: stairs. Most falls occur on the top step coming down from the landing, where lighting may create dangerous shadows or glare spots. Also, the change in lighting levels from room to room and particularly the dim light in hallways can cause falls on thresholds, rugs, and runners. Overall, it is important to keep stairs and hallways free of clutter and obstacles that can create safety hazards.

 ## Adaptations

▶▶ Make sure that lighting is uniform throughout hallways, with no dark or shadowy patches alternating with brightly lighted areas. Track lighting can help create even lighting levels.

▶▶ Make sure that stairs are well lighted, paying special attention to the top and bottom landings. Have additional lighting fixtures installed if necessary. If no other light is available, keep a flashlight in a convenient location at the top and bottom of the stairs.

▶▶ Mark the leading edge of the first and last steps of a staircase with bright paint or light-reflecting tape that contrasts with the background color of the flooring. If you use tape, be sure to change it frequently and keep it in good repair. It is helpful if the material on the leading edge is also textured, since this texture adds another sensory cue.

▶▶ Paint handrails in a bright color that contrasts with the walls and flooring. Handrails should be continuous and securely fastened on both sides of the staircase. Place a tactile mark on the handrail at the top and bottom of the staircase to remind you that the stairs are close by.

▶▶ Use solid, brightly colored hallway or stair runners to mark walking spaces clearly. Be sure to keep runners in good repair, since loose carpeting or frayed edges can create a safety hazard.

 ## Other Areas and Activities

The activities listed here may take place in any area of your home, but they are vital for maintaining an independent lifestyle. When you think about practical ways to carry out these activities, you need to consider safety needs first, and then lighting, contrast, color, and organization.

Telling Time

▶▶ If you have low vision, try using a large-print watch or clock that has either black numbers on a white

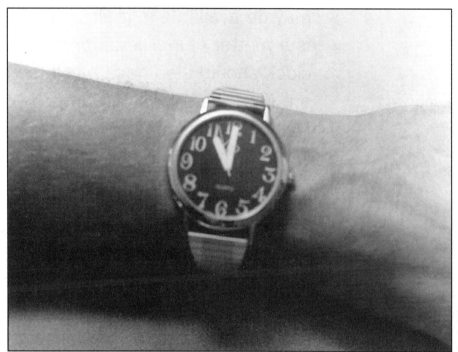

Andy Warren

A watch with large, clear numerals that contrast against the background can make telling time much easier.

background or white numbers on a black background. If you don't find a product that you like in a regular store, check independent living specialty catalogs. It is best if you select the watch or clock yourself, since individual preferences vary widely. A man's watch with a large face is usually a good choice. Some large-print watches are available with a choice of buckle or expansion bands; if you have arthritis or reduced sensation in your fingertips, an expansion band is usually a better choice.

▶▶ If you cannot see well enough to read large print, a talking watch or clock, available from specialty catalogs, can offer an alternative. As with a large-print watch or clock, it is best to make the selection yourself, since the controls may be small and difficult to manipulate, and the speaking voice may be available in male or female versions, which is a matter of individual preference. The watch or clock should also have a volume control. These are important considerations if you experience any type of hearing loss.

▶▶ A braille watch or clock is another alternative if you cannot read a large-print dial. This type of time-piece does not actually contain braille characters, but instead has an open face that allows you to feel a pattern of raised dots that substitute for numbers. These dots are placed at intervals around the watch or clock face; by using your fingertips, you can determine the position of the hands in relation to the raised dots. As with large-print watches, a man's watch with a large face is usually a better choice, since the dots are spaced farther apart and are easier to feel.

▶▶ If you purchase a wall clock, look for large, plain numbers or letters on a contrasting non-glare background. Try to position the clock at eye level, with sufficient floor space to allow you to stand as close as necessary to determine the time.

Identifying Coins and Bills

▶▶ To identify coins, remember that the penny and the nickel have smooth edges, while the dime, quarter, and half-dollar have rougher, milled edges that you can feel with your fingernail.

▶▶ To identify bills, try folding each denomination in a different way. For example, keep $1 bills flat, fold

$5 bills in half crosswise, fold $10 bills crosswise twice, and fold $20 bills in half lengthwise.

▶▶ Purchase a wallet or billfold with several different slots or pockets for sorting coins and bills, available in independent living catalogs.

▶▶ When you make a purchase, try to use bills and coins that are as close to the purchase price as possible. This way, you won't have to sort and identify your change when you return home.

Cleaning

▶▶ To make sure you don't miss any spots when you're cleaning tabletops or counters, follow a pattern of overlapping strokes and use your free hand as a guide. If the surface or floor area is large, divide it into sections with a tray or other marker or use pieces of furniture as landmarks.

▶▶ Store all your cleaning supplies in a bucket and carry it with you when you clean.

▶▶ Use an apron or a tote bag with large pockets for storing your cleaning supplies.

▶▶ Use a static duster or small, portable vacuum cleaner to collect dirt, instead of pushing the dirt from place to place as you dust or sweep.

▶▶ Wear an old pair of cotton gloves or socks over your hands for dusting.

▶▶ If you use a spray cleaner, locate the nozzle and spray directly into the cloth. This method is more accurate than spraying on to the surface.

▶▶ Clean windows in both vertical and horizontal patterns to avoid streaks.

▶▶ When you clean tabletops, hold a tray or cookie sheet at the front edge of the table, using a cloth to wipe toward the body and into the tray.

▶▶ When you vacuum or sweep, divide the floors into small sections, using furniture or other landmarks to outline the boundaries of your working area.

Home Maintenance

▶▶ Good lighting is essential for performing any type of home maintenance task. Install adjustable swing-arm and gooseneck lamps in all work areas or use a floor lamp on wheels that will allow you to move the light with you as you move around your work area.

▶▶ Consult your low vision specialist to determine if specific devices, such as a chest magnifier or a magnifier mounted on a flexible gooseneck stand, could help you with home maintenance tasks and whether they are appropriate for your needs and specific eye condition.

▶▶ Be sure to use safety goggles or glasses when performing any home maintenance task. Most types of safety glasses can be obtained with prescription lenses.

▶▶ Wrap contrasting tape around tool handles to make them easier to see and increase contrast with the work surface.

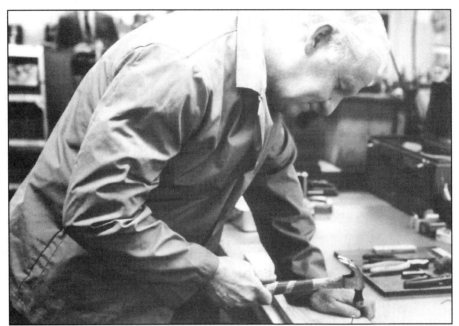

Susan Islam

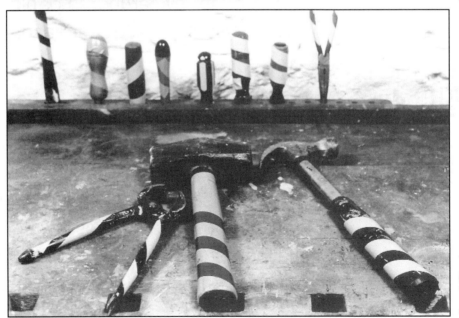

Janet Charles

Wrapping contrasting tape around tool handles makes them easier to see.

▶▶ Use color-coded bins to organize nails, screws, and sewing or craft supplies. Label each bin with any of the methods described in Chapter 2.

▶▶ Mark the handles of your frequently used tools with a Hi-Marks 3-D Marker, Spot 'n Line Pen, or other raised markings.

▶▶ Organize your tools, such as screwdriver sets or wrenches, by mounting them in order by size. Label your tools with any of the methods described in Chapter 2.

▶▶ For measuring, use a ruler with raised dots or lines, available from specialty catalogs, or mark a yardstick or tape measure with raised markings. You can also create your own templates by cutting pieces of sturdy cardboard or plastic to the lengths that you need to measure frequently.

 ## Just Outside the Door

The area where you enter and leave your home is an important part of your environment. Apartment buildings can pose special challenges to people with visual impairments because of their rows of identical doors and mailboxes and landings that all look the same when viewed from the elevator or stairway.

 ## Adaptations

▶▶ Have an emergency exit plan as well as an alternative plan in case of fire.

▶▶ Install a light fixture by the front door and replace burned-out lightbulbs promptly. In addition, consider installing lighting that contains a sensor to turn it on automatically when it detects motion or when it gets dark.

▶▶ If you use a doormat, make sure that it has a rubber backing to keep it from sliding.

▶▶ Identify your own apartment by hanging a large decorative wreath on your door or placing a few rubber bands around the doorknob.

▶▶ Apply a dot of Hi-Marks 3-D Marker, Spot 'n Line Pen, or other raised marking material to a specific spot on the door frame at your landing or elevator door to help you know when you've reached the right floor.

▶▶ To identify your mailbox in an apartment building, attach a piece of ribbon or a rubber band, apply a dot of raised marking material, or count how far your mailbox is from the end of the row of mailboxes.

☼ Everyday Activities

▶▶ To identify your keys, keep them in a specific order on your key chain, use colored keys, or place a colored rubber ring around the head of a particular key.

▶▶ To unlock your door, place your index finger alongside the keyhole to serve as a guide while you insert your key with the other hand.

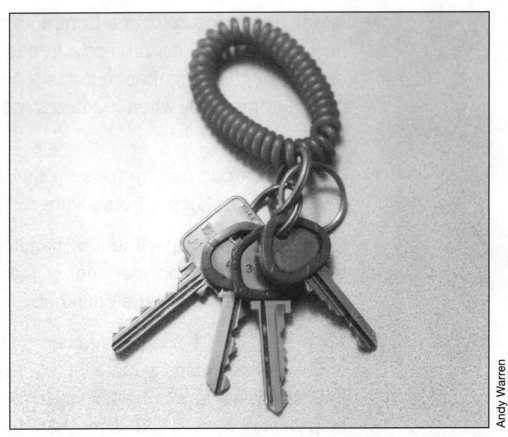

Andy Warren

Brightly colored rubber rings placed around the heads of different keys make them easier to distinguish.

As you walk around your home and consider the suggestions for each room that are offered here, you will undoubtedly think of ways to adapt them to your own particular living situation. You can start right away to put many of these ideas into use, and you will find that they can give you immediate help as you go about your everyday activities. You may come up with additional ideas later on as you become more familiar with the basic environmental principles and get used to the notion of adapting your surroundings or using adapted devices to make your life easier and safer. There is no better time to start than today.

Additional Health Conditions

Many older people who have experienced some vision loss also have another condition or disability that they need to consider when they think about making changes to their homes. Environmental modifications can also help older people with additional disabilities, as well as vision loss, to live independently and carry out their everyday activities more easily.

This chapter discusses simple adaptations that are helpful to older people with some of the most common disabilities—arthritis, cardiovascular disease, diabetes, hearing loss, Parkinson's disease, and complications from a stroke. If you have one or more of these conditions in addition to a visual impairment, consider the suggestions offered here in addition to those made elsewhere in this book. Many of the adaptations suggested in Chapters 2 and 3 can be useful in coping with these other conditions as well.

To find a rehabilitation professional who can help you learn more about adaptations that are appropriate for your combined vision loss and other disability, see "Where to Find Help" in Chapter 1. Most of the adaptive products mentioned in this chapter can be found in the independent living products catalogs listed in the Resource Guide at the back of this book, along with sources of more in-depth information and adaptations specifically designed for people with the conditions described in this chapter.

Arthritis

There are two main types of arthritis. *Rheumatoid arthritis* is a chronic inflammatory disease that primarily affects the joints and surrounding areas, causing stiffness and swelling of the wrists, fingers, knees, feet, and ankles and progressing toward the spine. It is accompanied by muscular degeneration and severe pain. It tends to flare up and subside unpredictably, leading to progressive, irreversible changes.

Osteoarthritis, or degenerative joint disease, results from years of accumulated wear and tear and usually affects the small joints in the fingers and toes, as well as the knees, hips, and spine. It is milder than rheumatoid arthritis, is usually noninflammatory, and is characterized by muscle weakness and joint pain. Regularly scheduled rest periods that relieve stress to the joints can be helpful in providing short-term relief from pain.

If you have either form of arthritis, pay special attention to the suggestions in Chapters 2 and 3 for getting organized, since good organization helps to minimize unnecessary activity, easing the burden on your joints. In addition, try the following:

■ Work for short periods, with planned rest periods in between. If you cook, keep a chair or stool near the stove, so you can rest whenever you need to.

■ Use a toaster, broiler oven, electric frying pan, crockpot, or microwave oven for tabletop cooking to eliminate bending over the stove and oven.

■ Arrange your storage facilities so the most frequently used items are placed within reach.

■ To relieve pressure on your finger joints, use pieces of contrasting colored foam tubing to build up utensil handles. Try using a rocker knife, available in independent living catalogs, to slice foods. As you rock the handle up and down, the sharp, curved blade slices through the food.

■ Use a rubberized or vinyl jar opener for gripping doorknobs and appliance controls.

■ Avoid lifting or carrying heavy household items. To transfer a pot from the counter to the stove, place the pot on a tray or cookie sheet with a raised rim and slide the tray along the counter instead of trying to lift the pot.

■ Use a cart with wheels to move items from room to room and to offer support while walking.

- When you read, support your book with a folding book stand instead of trying to hold it open.

- Install drawers on gliding tracks that open and close with a minimum of effort.

- Try not to start projects early in the morning when pain and stiffness are most pronounced. Sometimes a warm morning shower or bath can relieve joint pain. Be sure to use a bathtub bench or shower chair when bathing.

Cardiovascular Disease

Cardiovascular disease refers to conditions of both the heart and the blood vessels. The major risk factors are tobacco smoke, high blood cholesterol levels, high blood pressure, and physical inactivity. Diabetes, obesity, and individual response to stress can also contribute to the risk of heart disease. *Congestive heart failure* occurs when the heart is not pumping blood efficiently. Blood circulation is not normal, and fluid may gather in the body tissues, causing them to swell, especially in the feet and ankles.

When you think about adaptations for cardiovascular disease, it is important to concentrate on simplifying your everyday tasks and conserving energy. Suggestions in Chapters 2 and 3 for efficient organization will help in this regard. In addition, consider the following suggestions:

- Work for short periods, with planned rests in between. If you cook, keep a chair or stool near the stove so you can rest whenever you need to.

- Arrange your storage facilities so that the most frequently used items are placed within reach.

- Simplify cleanup by thinking ahead. Careful planning will enable you to use a minimum of utensils and dishes.

- To reduce cleanup time and conserve energy, use oven-to-tableware or serve directly from the pot. If you mix ingredients directly in a casserole dish, you can eliminate the need to wash extra bowls, dishes, and utensils.

- After preparing a meal, organize items that will need to be washed. Use a cart with wheels to bring dishes and pans to the work area and return them to cabinets and storage areas.

- Keep duplicates of cleaning supplies in different areas of your home to eliminate unnecessary walking from room to room.

- Use a long-handled dustpan to eliminate bending.

- Use a carpet sweeper or an electric broom instead of a heavier canister vacuum cleaner.

- Use an inexpensive back scratcher as a small reacher.

- Use grab bars in the tub area and next to the toilet and use a bathtub bench or shower chair when bathing.

Diabetes

Diabetes is a disease in which the body does not produce or properly use insulin, a hormone needed to convert sugar, starches, and other food into energy. The cause of diabetes is unknown, although both hereditary and environmental factors, such as obesity and lack of exercise, appear to play a part. There are two major types of diabetes. In Type 1, which occurs most often in children and young adults, the body does not produce any insulin. People with Type 1 diabetes must take daily insulin injections. Type 2 diabetes, the most common form of the disease, is a metabolic disorder resulting from the body's inability to make enough, or properly use, insulin. Type 2 diabetes accounts for 90 to 95 percent of the cases of diabetes.

The circulatory problems that accompany diabetes can cause an eye condition called *diabetic retinopathy,* in which damaged blood vessels in the retina leak blood components into the eye. This condition causes scattered blind spots, as well as blurred and changeable vision. Diabetes is the leading cause of new blindness in people aged 20–74 years of age.

One of the more common complications of diabetes, *diabetic neuropathy,* involves damage to the nerves throughout the body. This condition can reduce sensitivity in the hands and feet, cause cramping and pain, and affect balance. A support cane can be helpful when this occurs. Pay special attention to the safety tips in Chapters 2 and 3 to help minimize tripping hazards and prevent contact with hot substances. The following suggestions will also be helpful:

● Proper foot care is essential to prevent potentially serious infections. Therefore, wear comfortable, well-fitting shoes (not loose slippers) and good-quality socks to absorb moisture. Avoid socks with tight-fitting elastic tops that can impair circulation.

● Use a Caneseat to help you move throughout your home. This is a device that supports you like a cane, but has a folding seat attached to it that will provide relief when you need to rest.

● Use grab bars in the tub area and next to the toilet and use a bathtub bench or shower chair when bathing.

● Always wear shoes and socks when you sew. Use a magnet to collect any pins that may fall on the floor.

● Always use oven mitts when you are using the stove or oven and use padded potholders when you are handling a hot pan.

● Select kitchen utensils and tools with non-heat-conducting handles.

● Wear insulated rubber gloves when washing dishes by hand in hot water.

- Use an electronic liquid-level indicator (see Chapter 2) when you are pouring hot liquids.

- Label your diabetes medications with any of the methods described in Chapter 2.

- Contact your physician or a certified diabetes educator to learn more about adaptations for monitoring your blood glucose levels or measuring insulin.

Hearing Loss

Many older people mistakenly believe that hearing loss is a normal part of the aging process. They therefore may not investigate therapies, devices, and adaptations that might help reduce the impact of hearing loss, especially when it occurs in combination with vision problems. If you suspect that you may have a hearing loss, the first step is to have an evaluation and accurate diagnosis from an *audiologist,* a professional who specializes in this area, because correct evaluation and training is the key to using a hearing aid successfully. It is important to have realistic expectations, however, since hearing aids are not equally helpful for all types of hearing impairments.

If you have a hearing loss, you need to carefully consider the suggestions in Chapters 2 and 3 that relate to the use of sound or "talking" devices to see whether they will work for you. Also consider the following suggestions:

- Use an adapted watch or clock that vibrates instead of sounding a high-pitched alarm. Some vibrating alarm clocks are attached to a cord or sensor that you can place underneath your mattress.

- Most electronic liquid-level indicators vibrate as well as "whistle" when a liquid you are pouring reaches a spot near the rim of a glass or cup (see Chapter 2 for more information).

- Make sure that you can hear the signal or voice before you purchase any speaking or "talking" items.

- Turn a light on by the stove to remind you whenever you are using the stove or oven. Turn the light off only when you are finished.

- Reduce background noise as much as possible, including everyday household noises, such as the dishwasher, television, or washing machine. Most people with hearing loss have difficulty with conversations in this type of background noise.

- Pay special attention to proper lighting when you talk to other people. Even if your vision is severely reduced, it will still be easier to see facial expressions and gestures if you stand in good light and face the person with whom you are speaking.

- Use a telephone receiver that will amplify the speaker's voice.

Parkinson's Disease

Parkinson's disease is a slowly progressive degenerative condition, caused by the gradual loss of a small group of brain cells that control body movement. It usually develops in later life, with most individuals experiencing the first symptoms at age 40 or older. Signs and symptoms include muscle rigidity, lack of coordination, difficulty walking, impaired balance, a shuffling gait or dragging feet, a masklike facial expression, tremors, labored speech, and difficulty swallowing. The tremors usually affect the hands, although the head, tongue, and other muscles may be involved. Symptoms usually appear first in one hand, arm, or leg and gradually involve the entire body.

People with Parkinson's disease often have difficulty dressing, handling eating utensils, and performing personal hygiene tasks. They need to pay particular attention to the safety tips in Chapters 2 and 3 to help minimize tripping hazards. The following additional suggestions may be helpful:

● If you experience difficulty getting into and out of chairs, use a chair with solid arm rests. Also try placing two-inch blocks under the back legs of the chair, since a chair that is tipped forward slightly is easier to use.

● If possible, remove all doorsills throughout the home, since this is a primary cause of falls for individuals with Parkinson's disease.

● Handrails on staircases should be continuous and securely fastened on both sides.

● If you experience hand tremors, use an electric razor.

● Remove any accent or area rugs. They can be replaced with a floor mat with nonskid backing or wall-to-wall carpeting in a color that contrasts with the walls and fixtures.

● Use grab bars in the tub area and next to the toilet and use a bathtub bench or shower chair when bathing. If you need more support, use a toilet safety frame or a raised toilet seat.

● Lower the rods in your closets, so you don't have to reach too high for an item of clothing.

● Use a rocker knife for cutting and slicing. As you rock the handle up and down, the sharp, curved blade will slice through the food.

● If you eat slowly because swallowing is difficult, use an insulated dish to help keep food warm.

● Use a plate or food guard to keep food from falling off the edges of your plate.

Complications from a Stroke

A stroke is a disruption of the blood supply to, or within, the brain. If brain cells are injured or die from lack of oxygen or nutrients, the bodily functions controlled by those brain cells will be affected. Unlike other cells within the body, brain cells do not regenerate.

Disability from stroke can take many forms, depending on the area of the brain that is injured and the extent of the injury or damage to the brain tissue. Possible effects include paralysis or weakness on one side of the body, speech problems (aphasia), memory and reasoning problems, and fatigue. People who have experienced a stroke may also have difficulty controlling their emotions and may cry, curse, or laugh at inappropriate times.

When considering adaptations for a person who has had a stroke, pay special attention to suggestions about minimizing distracting visual clutter or confusion. You may have to make sure that adaptations can be used with one hand or on your better side. The following suggestions may also be helpful:

- When you cook, place utensils so they are arranged on your better side and are more convenient for a one-handed approach.

- To stabilize items, place a rubber pad, rubberized shelf liner, or a dampened sponge cloth under your mixing bowl or cutting board.

- Line your sink with a rubber mat to prevent glasses or dishes from breaking if you drop them.

- To open a jar with one hand, place the jar inside a drawer and lean against the drawer with your hip. The base of the jar will remain still while you turn the top.

- If you are using a one-handed can opener, place the can inside a pan before opening it to catch any spills.

- To transfer a pot from the counter to the stove, place the pot on a tray or cookie sheet with a raised rim and slide the tray instead of trying to lift the pot.

- Use a plate or food guard to keep food on your plate. If you have a reduced visual field on either side, remember to turn your plate a half turn after you finish eating to see if there is still food left on your plate.

- Use a one-handed rocker knife for cutting and slicing. As you rock the handle up and down, the sharp, curved blade will slice through the food.

- Keep work surfaces clear and free of clutter that can distract you. Use solid, nonpatterned tablecloths and place mats to minimize visual confusion and provide maximum contrast.

- Use grab bars in the tub area and next to the toilet and use a bathtub bench or shower chair when bathing. Use a pump bottle of liquid soap instead of a bar.

References

The following sources provided background information for this book:

Barker, P., Barrick, J., & Wilson, R. (1995). *Building sight: A handbook of building and interior design solutions to include the needs of visually impaired people.* London: Royal National Institute for the Blind.

Barker, P., & Bright, K. (1997). *A design guide for the use of colour and contrast to improve the built environment for visually impaired people.* London: Royal National Institute for the Blind.

Carlton, L. (1996). *Practical pointers for Parkinsonians.* Miami: National Parkinson Foundation.

Cooper, B. A. (1985). A model for implementing color contrast in the environment of the elderly. *American Journal of Occupational Therapy, 39*(4), 253–258.

Duffy, M. A. (1997). *New independence! Environmental adaptations in community facilities for adults with vision impairments.* Mohegan Lake, NY: Associates for World Action in Rehabilitation and Education (AWARE).

Edwards, L. E., Duffy, M. A., & Ray, J. S. (1998). The vision-related rehabilitation network. In R.L. Brilliant (Ed.), *Essentials of low vision practice.* Woburn, MA: Butterworth-Heineman.

Griffin-Shirley, N., & Groff, G. (1993). *Prescriptions for independence: Working with older people who are visually impaired.* New York: AFB Press.

Inkster, W., Newman, L., Weiss, D. S., & Yeadon, A. (1997). *Rehabilitation teaching for persons experiencing vision loss* (2nd ed.). New York: CIL Publications & Audiobooks.

Joffe, E. (1999). *A practical guide to the ADA and visual impairment.* New York: AFB Press.

Long, R. G. (1995). Housing design and persons with visual impairment: Report of focus-group discussions. *Journal of Visual Impairment & Blindness, 89*(1), 59–69.

McGillivray, R. (1984). *Aids and appliances review: Aids for elderly persons with impaired vision.* Boston: Carroll Center for the Blind.

Offner, R. (1994). *ADA accessibility guidelines: Provisions for people with impaired vision.* New York: The Lighthouse.

Orr, A. A. (1998). *Issues in aging and vision: A curriculum for university programs and in-service training.* New York: AFB Press.

Paskin, N., & Soucy-Moloney, L. A. (1994). *Whatever works.* New York: The Lighthouse.

Ponchillia P. E., & Ponchillia, S. V. (1996). *Foundations of rehabilitation teaching with persons who are blind or visually impaired.* New York: AFB Press.

Sicurella, V. J. (1977). Color contrast as an aid for visually impaired persons. *Journal of Visual Impairment & Blindness, 71*(6), 252–257.

Yeadon, A., Duffy, M. A., Geruschat, D., & Paskin, N. (1997). *New independence in the community: A self-help manual for community workers serving adults with vision impairments.* Mohegan Lake, NY: Associates for World Action in Rehabilitation and Education (AWARE).

Resource Guide

The information and suggestions presented in this book provide a good starting point for older people who are experiencing vision loss and their families to begin to make their lives more livable. For additional questions and needs readers are likely to have, however, there are a wide variety of resources that can be consulted. This Resource Guide lists a sample of the organizations and companies that offer assistance, information, referrals, products, and services related to vision loss and aging. If these organizations and companies do not have the answers to your questions, they will be able to refer you to a source that does.

For ease of use, this guide is divided into a few main sections: sources of information and referrals; sources of all kinds of products for independent living; sources of reading materials in various formats; sources of television programs and videotapes with video description; and sources of information about additional health conditions.

INFORMATION AND REFERRALS

The organizations listed in this section provide general information about visual impairment and blindness, eye conditions, and adapted or specialized

products and technology, as well as referrals for
additional information and services.

General Information
on Visual Impairment

American Academy of Ophthalmology

P.O. Box 7424
San Francisco, CA 94120 (415) 561-8500
Fax: (415) 561-8533
E-mail: comm@aao.org
www.eyenet.org

As the professional membership association for eye care
physicians, works to ensure that the public can obtain the best
possible eye care. Provides information on eye health for
consumers and referrals to member physicians.

American Foundation for the Blind

11 Penn Plaza, Suite 300
New York, NY 10001
(800) 232-5463 (800-AFB-LINE) or (212) 502-7600
Fax: (212) 502-7777
E-mail: afbinfo@afb.net
www.afb.org

Provides services to and acts as an information clearinghouse for
people who are blind and visually impaired and their families,
professionals, organizations, schools, and corporations.

Stimulates research and mounts program initiatives to improve
services to blind and visually impaired people. Publishes a wide
variety of professional, reference, and consumer books and
videos; the *Journal of Visual Impairment & Blindness (JVIB);
AccessWorld: Technology and People with Visual Impairments;* and
the *AFB Directory of Services for Blind and Visually Impaired
Persons in the United States and Canada.*

American Optometric Association

243 North Lindbergh Boulevard
St. Louis, MO 63141
(314) 991-4100
Fax: (314) 991-4101
www.aoanet.org

Provides information on visual conditions, eye diseases, and low vision; consumer guides for eye care; and referrals to optometrists in your area.

Hadley School for the Blind

700 Elm Street
Winnetka, IL 60093-0299
(800) 323-4238
Fax: 847-446-0855
E-mail: info@Hadley-School.org
www.hadley-school.org

Offers distance education courses for eligible students free of charge. Study areas include high school level courses and GEDs, academic courses, braille and communication skills, independent living, recreation and leisure, and technology.

Lighthouse International

111 East 59th Street
New York, NY 10022-1202
(800) 829-0500, (888) 222-9320,
    or (212) 821-9200 (consumer referral line)
TTY: (212) 821-9713
E-mail: info@lighthouse.org
www.lighthouse.org

Works to overcome visual impairment for people of all ages through worldwide leadership in rehabilitation services, education, research, and advocacy. Provides rehabilitation services, including training in adaptive living skills and computer skills for seniors. Publishes *Aging & Vision* newsletter and other publications on age-related vision loss for both professional and lay audiences. Maintains a catalog of products that are designed to make life easier for people with impaired vision.

National Association for Visually Handicapped

22 West 21st Street
New York, NY 10010
(212) 889-3141
Fax: (212) 727-2931
E-mail: staff@navh.org
or
3201 Balboa Street
San Francisco, CA 94121
(415) 221-3201
Fax: (415) 221-8754
E-mail: staffca@navh.org
www.navh.org

Provides information and referral for people with low vision on large-print books, low vision devices, medical advances and updates, craft materials and projects, resource guides, and religious materials. Sells low vision products and devices. Maintains a large-print mail-order library. Promotes public awareness of low vision.

Specific Eye Conditions

American Diabetes Association

1701 North Beauregard Street
Alexandria, VA 22314
(703) 549-1500 (local), (800) 342-2383, (888) 342-2383
    or (888) DIABETES (for referral to local offices)
Fax: (703) 549-6995
E-mail: customerservice@diabetes.org
www.diabetes.org

Provides information and public education about diabetes to consumers and professionals. Publishes books, journals, and brochures.

American Macular Degeneration Foundation

P.O. Box 515
Northampton, MA 01061-0515

(413) 268-7660

www.macular.org

Works for the prevention, treatment, and cure of macular degeneration by raising funds, educating the public, and supporting scientific research. Provides consumer information and referrals to eye care professionals.

American Society of Cataract and Refractive Surgery

4000 Legato Road, Suite 850

Fairfax, VA 22033

(703) 591-2220

Fax: (703) 591-0614

E-mail: ascrs@ascrs.org

www.ascrs.org

Provides information about cataracts and cataract and refractive surgery and referrals to ophthalmologists specializing in eye surgery.

Glaucoma Foundation

116 John Street, Suite 1605

New York, NY 10038

(212) 285-0080 or (800) GLAUCOMA (800-452-8266)

E-mail: info@glaucoma-foundation.org

www.glaucoma-foundation.org

Offers information and public education about glaucoma; provides free glaucoma screenings; funds research; and publishes consumer guides and brochures and *Eye to Eye,* a quarterly newsletter.

Other Useful Web Sites

AARP
(formerly *American Association of Retired Persons)*

www.aarp.org

Administration on Aging

U.S. Department of Health and Human Services

www.aoa.dhhs.gov

**Associates for World Action
in Rehabilitation and Education (AWARE)**

www.awareusa.org

Low Vision Council

www.lowvisioncouncil.org

Macular Degeneration Network

www.macular-degeneration.org

PRODUCTS FOR INDEPENDENT LIVING

General Independent Living Catalogs

The companies listed in this section sell by catalog a wide variety of specialized products that help people with visual impairments and other disabilities carry out everyday activities. The types of products in each catalog are indicated in the listing.

Ableware/Maddak

(973) 628-7600
Fax: (973) 305-0841
E-mail: custservice@maddak.com
Web site: www.maddak.com

Designer and manufacturer of assistive devices for activities of daily living. Offers adapted games, adapted scissors, eating utensils and tableware, enlarged grips, nonskid table mats, and writing devices.

American Printing House for the Blind

1839 Frankfort Avenue
P.O. Box 6085
Louisville, Kentucky 40206-0085
(502) 895-2405 or (800) 223-1839
Fax: (502) 899-2274

E-mail: catalogs@aph.org (request a catalog)
   or cs@aph.org (customer service)
www.aph.org

The Adult Life Products catalog features braille products, books, and supplies; large-print books; computer software and access products; labeling and marking products; lighting; low vision devices; mobility devices; personal care products; recreation and leisure products; talking products; and writing and reading devices.

Ann Morris Enterprises

551 Hosner Mountain Road
Stormville, NY 12582
(800) 454-3175 or (845) 227-9659
Fax: (845) 226-2793
www.annmorris.com

Braille products and supplies, adapted clocks and watches, computer software and access products, diabetes management products, kitchen and housekeeping items, labeling and marking products, lighting, low vision devices, mobility devices, personal care products, recreation and leisure products, talking products, telephones and accessories, and writing and reading devices.

Clotilde

Box 3000
Louisiana, MO 63353-3000
(800) 545-5002
E-mail: webmaster@clotilde.com
www.clotilde.com

Sewing notions, needle threaders, and regular and adaptive sewing supplies.

Independent Living Aids

200 Robbins Lane
Jericho, NY 11753
(800) 537-2118 or (516) 937-1848
Fax: (516) 937-3906

E-mail: can-do@independentliving.com
www.independentliving.com

Braille products and supplies, adapted clocks and watches, computer software and access products, diabetes management products, kitchen and housekeeping items, labeling and marking products, lighting, low vision devices, mobility devices, personal care products, recreation and leisure products, talking products, telephones and accessories, and writing and reading devices.

The Lighthouse Catalog

111 East 59th Street
New York, NY 10022-1202
(888) 770-7660
www.lighthouse.org and www.thelighthousecatalog.com

Adapted clocks and watches, diabetes management products, kitchen and housekeeping items, labeling and marking products, lighting, low vision devices, mobility devices, personal care products, recreation and leisure products, talking products, telephones and accessories, and writing and reading devices.

LS&S Group

P.O. Box 673
Northbrook, IL 60065
(800) 468-4789
TDD: (800) 317-8583
Fax: (847) 498-1482
E-mail: lssgrp@aol.com

Braille products and supplies, adapted clocks and watches, computer software and access products, diabetes management products, kitchen and housekeeping items, labeling and marking products, lighting, low vision devices, mobility devices, personal care products, recreation and leisure products, talking products, telephones and accessories, and writing and reading devices.

Maxi-Aids

42 Executive Boulevard
Farmingdale, NY 11735
(800) 522-6294 (orders) and (631) 752-0521 (information)

TTY: (631) 752-0738
Fax: (631) 752-0689
E-mail: sales@maxiaids.com
www.maxiaids.com

Braille products and supplies, adapted clocks and watches, computer software and access products, diabetes management products, kitchen and housekeeping items, labeling and marking products, lighting, low vision devices, mobility devices, personal care products, recreation and leisure products, talking products, telephones and accessories, and writing and reading devices.

Braille Products

See "General Independent Living Catalogs" for information about aluminum clothing tags, braille labeling guns, labeling tape, money braillers, overlays for appliance dials, braille watches and clocks, and all types of braille reading materials, including cookbooks.

Lighting Products

The companies listed here specialize in products that can help improve the lighting in your home. See also "General Independent Living Catalogs" for other sources of lighting, lamps, and lightbulbs, including swing-arm lamps, combination fluorescent-incandescent lamps, magnifying lamps, halogen lamps and bulbs, Chromalux bulbs, full-spectrum bulbs, and compact fluorescent bulbs.

A.L.P. Lighting Components

6333 Gross Point Road
Niles, IL, 60714-3915
(773) 774-9550

Fax: (773) 774-9331
E-mail: info@alp-ltg.com
www.alp-ltg.com

Manufacturer of a wide variety of lighting fixtures, lamps, lightbulbs, louvers, reflectors, and compact fluorescent bulbs.

Dazor Manufacturing Corporation

4483 Duncan Avenue
St Louis, MO 63110
(800) 345-9103 or (314) 652-2400
Fax: (314) 652-2069
E-mail: info@dazor.com
www.dazor.com

Manufacturer of a wide variety of task lights and lamps, including swing arm, combination fluorescent/incandescent, halogen, and magnifying.

Philips Lighting Company

200 Franklin Square Drive
Somerset, NJ 08875-6800
(800) 555-0050 or (732) 563-1731
Fax: (732) 563-3740
www.lighting.philips.com

Manufacturer of a wide variety of lightbulbs, including fluorescent, compact fluorescent, incandescent, halogen, and full spectrum. Also provides specialty lighting and innovative lighting solutions.

Products for Labeling

The companies listed here specialize in products for labeling and identification. See also "General Independent Living Catalogs" for other sources of products for labeling and marking, including clothing identifiers, Hi-Marks 3-D Marker, Spot 'n Line Pen, prescription labels, raised marks and dots, marking pens and materials, and audio talk labels.

Talking Prescription Labels

Rx Partners Pharmacy

500 Old Pond Road, Suite 403
Bridgeville, PA 15017
(888) 477-6337
www.rxpartnerspharmacy.com

Distributor of Aloud, an audio prescription labeling system.

Millennium Compliance Corporation

P.O. Box 649
Southington, CT 06489
(860) 426-0542
www.talkingrx.com

Distributor of Talking Rx, an audio prescription labeling system.

Marking, Labeling, and Identification Products

Gladys E. Loeb Foundation

2002 Forest Hill Drive
Silver Spring, MD 20903-1532
(301) 434-7748 (telephone or fax)

Manufacturer of Loeb's Labels, durable plastic nonbraille food-shaped labels mounted on durable elastic bands.

Seton Identification Products

Department AR-11
20 Thompson Road
P.O. Box 819
Branford, CT 06405-0819
(800) 243-6624
www.seton.com

Safety signs, safety labels, sign and label machines, reflective tape, warning tape, marking materials, and large-print letters.

READING

The sources listed here provide reading materials in alternate formats, including large-print, braille, or recordings. See also "General Independent Living Catalogs" for products that can help with reading, such as closed-circuit television systems, computer adaptations, computer hardware and software, and additional large-print reading materials, including cookbooks.

Choice Magazine Listening

P.O. Box 10
Port Washington, NY 11050
(516) 883-8280
Fax: (516) 944-6849

A free monthly anthology of current articles chosen from over 100 leading magazines. Recorded in four-track Library of Congress format. Distributed free through regional libraries. Also available through individual subscription.

CIL Publications and Audiobooks

500 Greenwich Street, 3rd floor
New York, NY 10013
(888) CIL-8333
Fax: (212) 219-4078
E-mail: cilpubs@visionsvcb.org
www.cilpubs.com

Offers self-study audiotapes and audiobooks for people who are blind and visually impaired. Subjects include indoor mobility, personal management, and sensory development.

Doubleday Large Print Home Library

6550 East 30th Street
P.O. Box 6309

Indianapolis, IN 46206-6309
(371) 541-8920

Offers a large-print Book-of-the-Month Club.

International Association of Audio Information Services

(800) 280-5325
http://iaais.org

An international organization of radio reading services that provides audio access to information for people who are print disabled (blind, visually impaired, learning disabled, or physically disabled), including news, feature stories, sports, advertisements, and other special programs. Connects listeners with services in their area.

In Touch Networks

15 West 65th Street
New York, NY 10023
(212) 769-6270

Provides national programming services for local radio reading services for people who are blind and visually impaired. Offers closed circuit radio broadcasts of national and local newspapers and magazines.

Matilda Ziegler Magazine for the Blind

20 West 17th Street
New York, NY 10011
(212) 242-0263

Publishes the *Matilda Ziegler Magazine for the Blind,* a free monthly general-interest periodical. Provided in braille and on cassette.

National Library Service for the Blind and Physically Handicapped

Library of Congress
1291 Taylor Street, NW
Washington, DC 20011
(202) 707-5100 or (800) 424-8567
TDD: (202) 707-0744

Fax: (202) 707-0712
E-mail: nls@loc.gov
http://lcweb.loc.gov/nls

Provides a free library service for people who are unable to read standard print materials because of a visual or physical impairment. Recorded Talking Books and magazines and braille publications are delivered to eligible borrowers by postage-free mail and through a network of cooperative libraries. Also distributes Talking Book machines.

New York Times Large Type Weekly

229 West 43rd Street
New York, NY 10036
(800) 631-2580 (information and subscriptions)
www.nytimes.com

Publishes a weekly news summary from the *New York Times*.

Reader's Digest Fund for the Blind

P.O. Box 241
Mount Morris, IL 61054
800-877-5293 (information and subscriptions)
www.readersdigest.com

Offers selections from *Reader's Digest, Reader's Digest* condensed books, and other *Reader's Digest* publications.

VIDEO DESCRIPTION

Some television programs and films on videotape are available in video-described versions; that is, they have explanations and descriptions of the visual elements inserted on the sound track without interfering with the sounds and dialogue that are part of the program. For some television programs, these descriptions can be heard on a separate audio channel that is available on most stereo televisions sold in the United States, called Secondary Audio Program or SAP. Programs are available on many public broadcasting and cable stations, and video-described movies can be purchased or borrowed from some libraries and video stores.

Descriptive Video Service: Media Access Group at WGBH

125 Western Avenue
Boston, MA 02134
617-300-3600 (local) or 800-333-1203 (prerecorded information only)
Fax: (617) 300-1020
E-mail: access@wgbh.org
www.wgbh.org/access

Narrative Television Network (NTN)

5840 South Memorial Drive, Suite 312
Tulsa, OK 74145-9082
(918) 627-1000 or (800) 801-8184
Fax: (918) 627-4101
E-mail: webmaster@narrativetv.com
www.narrativetv.com

ADDITIONAL HEALTH CONDITIONS

The organizations listed in this section can provide more information on conditions other than vision loss through books, magazines, brochures, catalogs, and web sites, as well as through referral to local chapters and self-help groups. Also listed here are distributors of independent living products specifically designed for individuals with these additional conditions.

Arthritis

Arthritis Foundation

1330 West Peachtree Street
Atlanta, Georgia 30309
(800) 283-7800
www.arthritis.org

Ableware/Maddak

(973) 628-7600
Fax: (973) 305-0841
E-mail: custservice@maddak.com
Web site: www.maddak.com

Designer and manufacturer of assistive devices for activities of daily living. Offers adapted games, adapted scissors, eating utensils and tableware, enlarged grips, nonskid table mats, and writing devices.

Cardiovascular Disease

American Heart Association

7272 Greenville Avenue
Dallas, TX 75231
(800) AHA-USA-1 or (800) 242-8721
www.americanheart.org

Diabetes

American Diabetes Association

1701 North Beauregard Street
Alexandria, VA 22314
(703) 549-1500 (local), (800) 342-2383, (888) 342-2383
    or (888) DIABETES (for referral to local offices)
Fax: (703) 549-6995
E-mail: customerservice@diabetes.org
www.diabetes.org

Hearing Loss

American Academy of Audiology

8300 Greensboro Drive, Suite 750
McLean, Virginia 22102
(800) AAA-2336 or (703) 790-8466
Fax: (703) 790-8631
www.audiology.org

Hearmore Products

42 Executive Boulevard
Farmingdale, NY 11735
(800) 881-4327
TTY: (631) 752-3277
Fax: (631) 752-0689
E-mail: sales@hearmore.com
www.hearmore.com

Distributes products for people with hearing impairments, including alert systems, door sensors, smoke detectors, adapted clocks and watches, telephone amplifiers, adapted telephone systems, TTY and TDD systems, computer software and access, products for people who are deaf-blind.

Parkinson's Disease

American Parkinson Disease Association

1250 Hylan Boulevard, Suite 4B
Staten Island, NY 10305-1946
(718) 981-8001 or (800) 223-2732
Fax: (718) 981-4399
E-mail: info@apdaparkinson.org
www.apdaparkinson.org

Stroke

American Stroke Association

7272 Greenville Avenue
Dallas, TX 75231

(888) 4-STROKE or (888) 478-7653

www.strokeassociation.org

National Stroke Association

9707 E. Easter Lane

Englewood, CO 80112

(800) STROKES or (303) 649-9299

Fax: (303) 649-1328

www.stroke.org

Ableware/Maddak

(973) 628-7600

Fax: (973) 305-0841

E-mail: custservice@maddak.com

www.maddak.com

Designer and manufacturer of assistive devices for activities of daily living. Offers adapted games, adapted scissors, eating utensils and tableware, enlarged grips, nonskid table mats, and writing devices.

About
Maureen A. Duffy

Maureen A. Duffy, M.S., RTC, is Director of the Master of Science and Certificate Programs in Rehabilitation Teaching, and Assistant Professor, Department of Graduate Studies in Vision Impairment, at the Institute for the Visually Impaired, Pennsylvania College of Optometry, in Elkins Park. As a member of the Advisory Board of Associates for World Action in Rehabilitation and Education (AWARE) and of their Central European Project, she assisted in the development of gerontological content for the Polish-American Postgraduate Teacher Training Program in Rehabilitation Teaching and Orientation and Mobility at Akademia Pedagogiki Specjalnej im. Marii Grzegorzewskiej (Maria Grzegorzewska Academy of Special Education), Warsaw, Poland, where she is an adjunct faculty member. Ms. Duffy is a certified rehabilitation teacher and previously worked at a number of community agencies.

Ms. Duffy has written and edited a number of books, chapters, and articles about the needs of older people with vision loss, here as well as in Poland, and has presented many papers and workshops at conferences in the United States and abroad. She is currently President of Division 11 (Rehabilitation Teaching) of the Association for Education and Rehabilitation of the Blind and Visually Impaired (AER) and received the 1999-2000 Educator of the Year Award from the Department of Graduate Studies, Pennsylvania College of Optometry.